PRAISE FOR *FOOTSTEPS TO SUCCESS*

"This book is amazingly inspirational. I have had the pleasure of photographing both Jennifer Nicole Lee and Carolin Mildner. They have unmatchable charisma, beauty, charm, wit, and pizzazz. And now this joint book from them is a must buy if you want to add energy and happiness to your lifestyle!"

—Rula Kanawati, Celebrity Photographer
www.RulaKanawatiPhotography.com

"Written by JNL, the creator of the JNL Fusion workout method, and Carolin Mildner, one of our top JNL Fusion master trainers, this book gives you a double whammy of motivation. After reading this book, you will walk away with a new, fresh perspective of what is possible in your life. I recommend this book to everyone who wants to live their best life possible."

—Janis Saffel, Chief Officer of Business Development for JNL
Worldwide, Inc.
www.JanisSaffell.com

"Both JNL and Carolin have immeasurable passion. As a mom and wife myself, I know and understand firsthand what a challenge it is to juggle all of our mom and wife duties while still trying to stay in shape and enjoy living a fun, fit lifestyle as a family. Get this book—you will recharge your mind, body, and spirit to never give up!"

—Adita Lang, Director of JNL Fusion Workout Education
www.NutritionalBrilliance.com

"Do you have your own big goal? Now the only thing you need is the essential knowledge about the 'how'! You get it all in this very special book from two very hard-working, dedicated, lovely, and successful women—Jennifer Nicole Lee and my fantastic wife Carolin Mildner. You carry your own future in your hands now! Don´t waste time but read, train, live, and repeat these valuable contents and you will get back success in all areas of life! Use this bible for your endless potential in an ideal way for you. Start here. Start now. Turn the page and become the person you want to be. Learn to turn on and be yourself!"

—Andreas Konstantin Mildner, founder and senior partner of Mildner & Associates, entrepreneur and business speaker, known as "the hardest rhetoric trainer of Germany"

FOOTSTEPS TO SUCCESS:

HOW TO BE FIT AND SUCCESSFUL IN ALL AREAS OF YOUR LIFE

Jennifer Nicole Lee and Carolin Mildner

Front cover photo by Rula Kanawati
Back cover photo by Alex Gonzalez

ISBN: 0615994342
ISBN 13: 9780615994345

Jennifer Nicole Lee Worldwide Media Group

**For more healthy-lifestyle programs
and information, please visit:**

www.JNLMethod.com
www.CarolinMildner.com
www.JNLWorldwide.net
www.JNLEuroConference.com

DEDICATION FROM JENNIFER NICOLE LEE

I would like to dedicate this book first and foremost to my creator, God, for giving me the strength to write this book, that it may empower and motivate all who read it. I also want to thank my husband and sons for always believing in me and supporting me with endless love. I want to thank all of my JNL Fitness family worldwide! You are so encouraging and eager to learn and be the best! Special thanks to all of my certified JNL Fusion trainers and master trainers, who are now following my Footsteps to Success! And big thanks to our number-one JNL Fusion master trainer in all of Germany, Carolin Mildner. Your weight-loss success story and strength inspire us all!

I believe in *you*!

Jennifer Nicole Lee

Best-Selling Author, International Fitness Icon, Top Super Fitness Model, Creator of the JNL Fusion Workout Method

DEDICATION FROM CAROLIN MILDNER

For me, writing this book is a dream come true. I am so thankful and honored that I have been able to share my weight-loss transformation in this book with all of you! My biggest role model is Jennifer Nicole Lee, as she helped me to realize that I, too, could lose weight, get in shape, and enjoy my life again after becoming a mom. She is my highest inspiration and motivation from the beginning of my weight-loss success story to the end. First, I would like to dedicate this book to JNL because she gave me strength every day. JNL helped me to believe in myself and to never give up on fighting for my dreams. Also, I can't say thank you enough for what she did for me through her hard work and loving spirit for our JNL Fusion fitness family worldwide. She has created an international JNL Fusion fitness family whose members support each other, and with her and them I can reach the stars!

I also want to thank my wonderful husband for all his support. I am so grateful that he believes in me and is always there rooting me on to my next level of success. And also a big, warm, special thank-you to my two beautiful sons! They are the big reasons *why* I work so hard to achieve my goals and also why I think big in life. And big thanks to my JNL Fusion family! When other women are negative and jealous of each other, we are rocking and succeeding together. My JNL Fusion sisters and fitness family, you all showed me what I can achieve in life and to live my dreams!

Carolin Mildner

JNL Fusion Master Trainer, Personal Trainer, Weight-Loss Success Story, IFBB Fitness Figure Athlete

JENNIFER NICOLE LEE

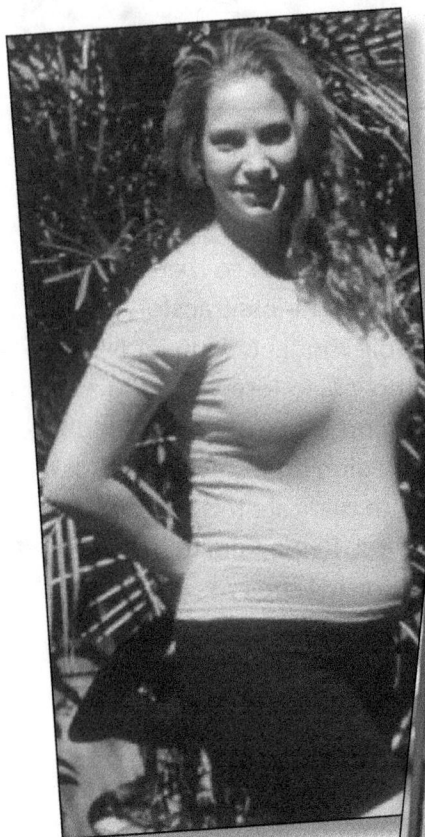

BEFORE

AFTER

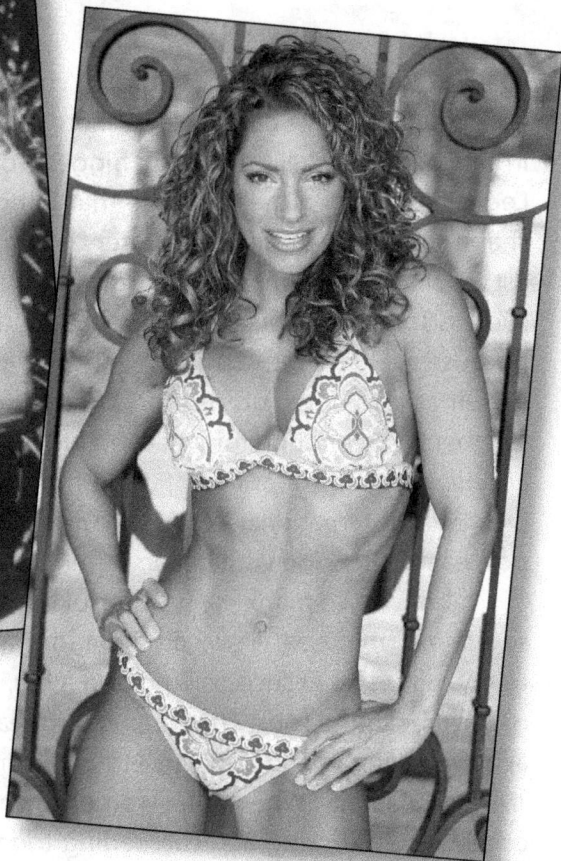

JNL

JENNIFER NICOLE LEE
WORLDWIDE

CAROLIN MILDNER

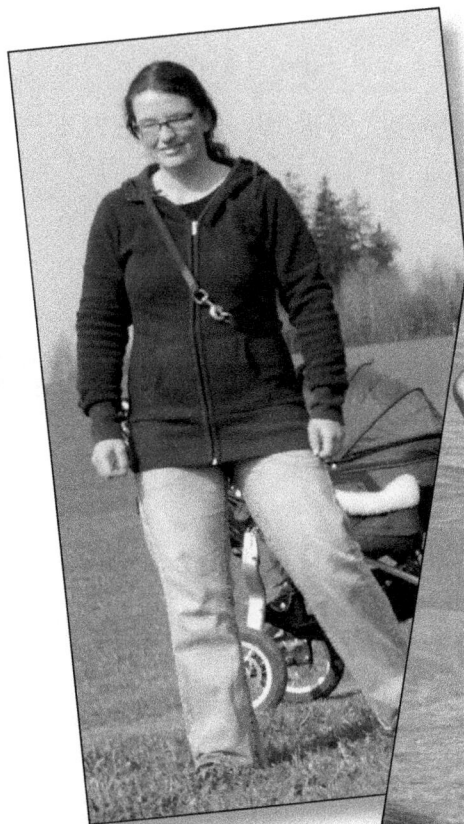

BEFORE

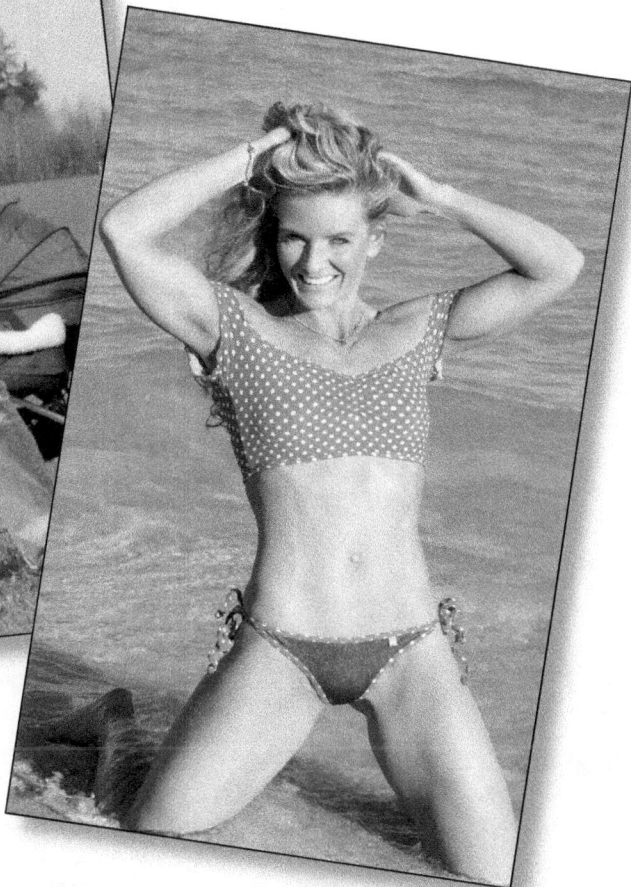

AFTER

CM

CAROLIN MILDNER

TABLE OF CONTENTS

Chapter 6

Chapter 7

Chapter 8

Chapter 9

FOREWORD

When Jennifer and Carolin asked me to write the foreword to this book, I was so honored. This book is a life changer for all who read it. Having known and worked with both Jennifer Nicole Lee and Carolin Mildner has been such a huge blessing. Both of these women are powerhouses! They share the same amazing story! Two women, yet one powerful message! It was Jennifer's inspirational weight-loss success story that helped motivate Carolin to also take positive action in her own life. They both lost over seventy pounds leading them to become highly sought after fitness and weight-loss experts known worldwide!

I urge all to read this book. Not only will you walk away with a better understanding of what the "Footsteps to Success" are, but you will have the newfound motivation to go after your own weight fitness goals and dreams!

As a red carpet celebrity photographer, my job and lifestyle is very busy and extremely demanding. So I want the right info, from people who I can trust! Many can get lost in the fitness industry with all of the fad diets and extreme exercising. So this book is an excellent, complete lifestyle guide that will get you results—FAST! I love the straightforwardness and honest, clear message that both of these fitness experts provide. They are rooting for your success! They want you to achieve your fitness goals, because as they say, "your success is their success"!

Warmly,

Rula Kanawati

Red Carpet Celebrity Photographer

www.RulaKanawatiPhotography.com

Chief Photographer for Fitness Model Factory

www.FitnessModelFactory.com

ACKNOWLEDGMENTS

from Jennifer Nicole Lee and Carolin Mildner

We want to thank all who helped in making this dream a reality. This manuscript is now a book being sold worldwide, and we could not have done it without your help!

Special recognition goes to celebrity photographer, Rula Kanawati, who is one of the most wonderful people in this world! Your big heart and spirit warm everyone you meet!

Thank you to Janis Saffell, our chief director of business development. Your professionalism, vision, and focus are unmatchable!

Special thanks to our director of education, Adita Lang. Your big heart, true friendship, and expansive experience in the fitness industry always amaze us!

And a huge congratulations to you who are reading this right now! We believe that there are no such things as accidents, and that everything happens for a reason. The fact that you are reading this means that you're finally ready to say good-bye to the old you and say hello to the new, improved you that you were always meant to be.

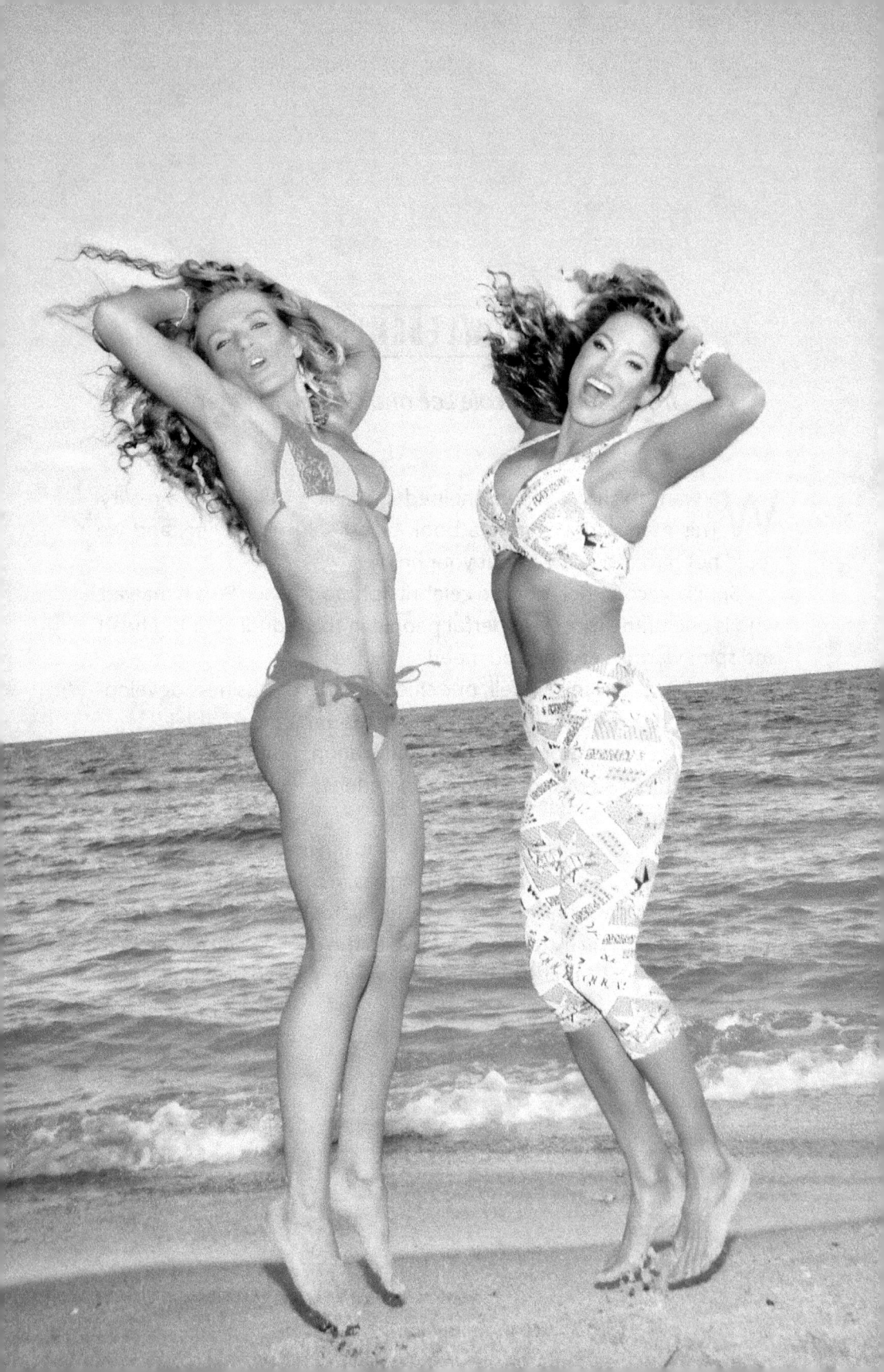

THE FOOTSTEPS TO SUCCESS

1. Know exactly what you want! How do you want look? How do you want to feel?

2. Find your Big *Why*! What is *your WHY*? Why do want to lose weight? Why now and not next year? What are your motivations?

All your motivations have to come from you and not come from your husband, neighbors, friends, and family! You have to change for you because *you* are the most important person in your world.

3. Believe in yourself and love yourself! Tell yourself you can and you will! Be proud of who you are and love yourself just like you are now. Love your body how it is right now—even if you are not at your goal weight or fitness level.

4. Set your detailed goals—and also a time frame. Your goals has to be big but reachable—one step at a time. Set a date for your BIG end goal and breakdown your in-between goals footstep by footstep. In other words, reverse engineer your actions from the deadline goal date. This is the direction to your goal! If you have no direction from *where* to *there*, you can't step in the footsteps of others who have reached their goals. If you have your detailed goals, route, and your small targets, you can find your role model! And we both wish so much that you decide to go in the footsteps that we show you in this special book!

5. TAKE ACTION! Not tomorrow. Not next week. Not next month. *NOW!* Go to the grocery store and get healthy and delicious options to reach your goals! Make your own schedule for the activities that bring you to your biggest wishes.Don´t just read this book, *live* it! Read it, work it, live it, and enjoy the journey.

6. Stay on track on the footsteps to success and never give up! Sometimes you will have hard times, and it can be very difficult to stay on track. We are humans. We make mistakes, but we never forget the lessons we learn. If you know this from the beginning, it will be much easier to stay on track! Winners never quit. Giving up is no option. Learn from your faults, get up, put your crown in the right direction, and go forward!

7. Eat five to six little healthy meals per day. Nutrition is about 70 percent of your weight loss success!

8. Work out smarter, not harder! Most of women train endlessly on cardio machines, but without any results! Use the JNL FUSION method and you will see very quick amazing results—you will love it because it will give you lifelong results fast! Do your workout in the morning with weights to build sexy and sleek muscles and you will speed your metabolism like a fat burning machine!

9. Rinse and Shine! Our bodies are up to 70 percent water. Drink a minimum of three liters water per day and your body will flush out all of its toxins. If you are always hydrated, you will "pee off the pounds." When you are thirsty, your body sometimes mistakens this as being hungry, so you will keep false hunger pangs away.

10. Schedule in your downtime, rest, and relaxation.
Muscle is built while you are sleeping, not awake. So rest, and make sure you always get a good night's rest. Your body needs one to two days off from training.

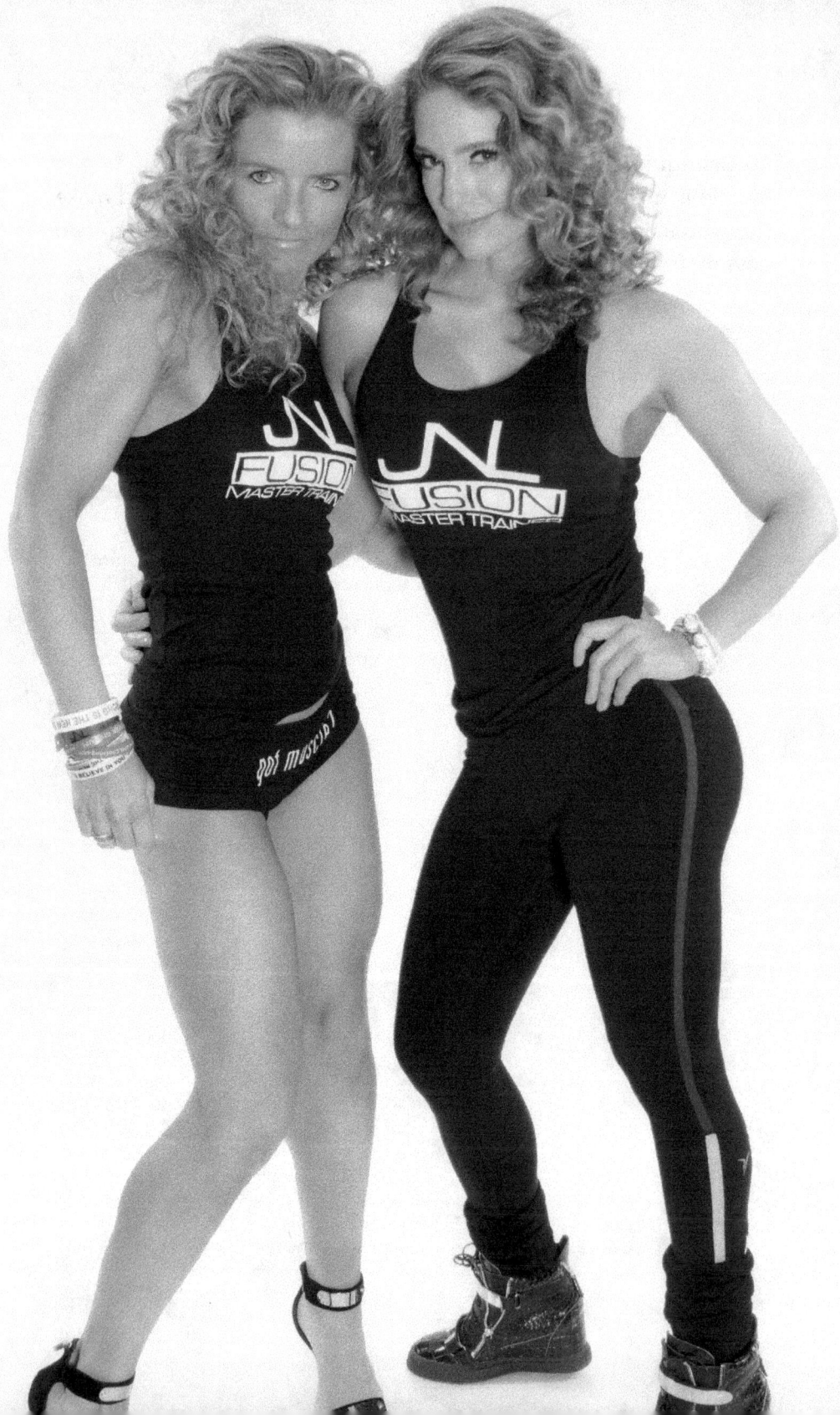

CHAPTER 1

Introduction: Our Personal Weight-Loss Success Stories and What You Can Learn From Us

C ongratulations on making a wise decision to invest in yourself, your health, and your fitness future. It's obvious that you want to change something in your life, and the great news is that we are here to help you. So get ready for a fun, fit ride! Say good-bye to the old you and hello to the new, fit, and healthy you.

After reading this fit-lifestyle guide you will:

- Know how to increase your metabolism with simple tips and tools
- Exercise smarter, not harder
- Know our favorite fundamental weight-training exercises
- Learn the difference between good and bad carbs and fats
- Understand that fitness must start in your mind
- Learn how fiber is your best friend when it comes to weight loss
- Learn how not to get bored or discouraged when hitting a plateau
- Break through mental and physical barriers that keep you from achieving your goals

We know the weight-loss journey very well, as we each lost over seventy pounds after the birth of our children, leading us to become fitness competitors and true weight-loss experts. Therefore, we both know the Footsteps to Success that will get you to your goal more quickly and easily. And we are also here to root for you along the journey to your ultimate fitness level. We don't want you to go through the detours, the obstacles, and the dead ends that many experience on their weight-loss and fitness journeys. We are here to help you create a success plan, cheer for you along the way, and help you win in the game of weight loss!

Yes, there are many so-called experts in the fitness, wellness, and weight-loss industry. This market is extremely oversaturated with fad diets from people who either are not in shape or have never had a problem with being overweight.

This is why our book is different. You see, both of us have been overweight and have gone through the weight challenges of being pregnant and having children very close in age back to back. We not only got in good shape after giving birth but also got into superfit competition shape with award-winning physiques and physical conditions. We are not "preaching from the pulpit" but speaking from our own true experiences and sharing our Footsteps to Success that will also work for you!

Also, the fitness and weight-loss industry is riddled with countless "miracle" products such as weight-loss pills, slimming creams, and other scams. Many people buy into these quick-fix products, and the only thing they exercise is their wallet! We don't want you to be fooled. Many companies just want your money and then move on to the next customer once they get it. They don't really care if you lose weight or not. But we are different in that we truly care and are compassionate toward you. We know that your success is our success. We are women who lost weight the safe and natural way and have kept the weight off for good. We want to spare you stress, anger, and frustration, and we really do want you to make improvements in your life and follow the Footsteps to Success. We lost our weight while raising children, working, taking care of our households, and also being loving, dedicated wives and moms. We didn't use excuses or give up. So we are here to support you and to help you be strong when you feel weak—so you, too, will never give up or give in when it comes to achieving your weight-loss goals.

Ask yourself this question: How nice would it be if you had a GPS to give you directions through this wild jungle of confusing fitness advice, gimmicks, and tricks? Would you appreciate having a map you could follow that would lead you straight to your desired outcome? Or how great would it be if you found step-by-step instructions that led you right to where you wanted to be in life?

Well, this is exactly what you have in your hands. Not only will you enjoy great workout tips and nutritional information but also inspiration to help to keep you motivated. We invite you to follow in our footsteps in carving out your own personal road to success!

My Story by Jennifer Nicole Lee

I grew up poor with very humble beginnings. I yo-yoed up and down on the scale and tried fad diets my entire life—until I become a mom. After the birth of my children, I made the decision to stop following in the footsteps of all the women who became mothers, gained weight, and became unhappy and miserable. I decided instead to follow in the footsteps of other women who were in shape and happy and lived lives full of joy! I still can't believe that I have appeared on over seventy magazine covers, have authored and published over six books, and also am an internationally recognized fitness celebrity. I'm thrilled to say that I lost over seventy pounds and have kept the weight off through my accredited JNL Fusion workout method, which I created.

My story of yo-yo dieting and my love/hate relationship with food is a long one! But I've learned from it to do the right things, so I humbly share it with you so you, too, will learn what to do and what not what to do!

"So what do you want to eat today?" This was my Italian family's favorite question! My mom and dad, being true Italians, bombarded my two older sisters, my younger brother, and me with food constantly.

This food-focused question was the first thing I was asked when I woke up. Every morning it was a serious topic of discussion over a fattening breakfast of fried eggs and sausage prepared with love by Mom. Sometimes, discussions over what the day's menu would end in a heated debate: my sister wanted lasagna while my brother wanted spaghetti, meatballs, and sausage. Eating was an all-day affair with no breaks! And no matter what I said, it was coming my way, and large portions of it!

Needless to say, my mom and dad showed their love for us through food. Well, what do you expect from an Italian family? The use of food as a medium for love was passed down from generation to generation, and it was the only thing they knew how to do.

Not only that, but I inherited the "fat gene." The correct medical term would be a "slow metabolism." My slow metabolic rate further worsened because I was constantly surrounded by poor food choices and large portions. Growing up, I gained and stored weight so easily. Do you ever feel sometimes that all you have to do to gain five pounds is just look at a piece of chocolate cake? Well, that was me! We were always eating. My days consisted of one large, never-ending meal. And we ate for every occasion.

Perhaps I should rephrase that by saying we did not "eat" but rather "pigged out" and "feasted." When we were happy, we would celebrate and eat. When we were sad, we would mourn and eat. When we were bored, we would eat. And when we were planning a special occasion, we would surround the event with food. It was always about food and what the next meal was.

Even after my parents separated, they graduated to "food wars." My mom would constantly ask me, "So whose lasagna is better, mine or your father's?" My dad would seem a little peeved if we went to his house on a full stomach from our mom's. He would ask, "So what did she feed you?" It seemed as though he was strategizing a plan to one-up her at his next meal.

I was brainwashed, if you will, with the idea that food was truly the end all! And boy, did I yo-yo. The only fitness knowledge I had growing up was the starvation diet. I knew that I had to lose weight, but the only thing I did to accomplish that was either not eat much or simply not eat at all. My body hoarded the fat pounds instead of losing them. And we have all been there—from Oprah Winfrey and her liquid diet to Princess Diana and her bouts of bulimia to many of today's celebrities going stick skinny and many of my clients having used "unhealthy" means to get "healthy." It is a crazy diet cycle that may have helped us temporarily lose weight but in the end only lets us gain it all back, or more, after the diet ends!

Have you ever felt like a gerbil running on one of those stationary wheels, going nowhere fast? That's what the endless unhealthy cycle of losing and gaining feels like. But with our Footsteps to Success lifestyle program, your outcome will be different! With FTS you will transform your body into a fat-burning machine, unlocking your fat-burning and weight-loss potential because we will take you to the core of the problem: your metabolic rate.

In this miraculous book you will learn so many tools that you will be soon carrying with you a bag of tricks you can use at any time. I like to call it "having ammunition to fight fat!" I drastically changed all the associations I had been taught about food into positive tools I used in Footsteps to Success. In doing so, I was able to transform my body into a fat-burning machine, unlocking my weight-loss potential by primarily stoking my metabolic rate.

The "Aha!" Moment That Changed My Life

I knew I was out of shape, but I could not imagine I looked that *bad*! It was an ordinary summer day, but it changed my life forever. I will never forget it. It was mid-May, official swimsuit season. I had a friend brave enough to take a picture of me in a fuchsia bikini. I didn't know it at the time, but this is my famous "before" picture.

After my brave and willing friend took the snapshot, I glanced at it. And then *it* happened. It was my "aha!" moment. I couldn't believe my eyes. Was that me? What had happened; where had I gone? I did not recognize myself. I knew I was out of shape, but did I look that bad? Yes,

I knew that I was masking my weight by wearing baggy black clothes, lots of makeup, and big hair. But I stripped my daily costume away and placed myself in a bikini to get real. And boy, did I get real with myself.

From that point on, I did all I could to lose the weight and get in shape. I placed that photograph in my bathroom so I could see it every day when I got ready in the morning. I saw it at night before I took my shower. There wasn't a day that I didn't look at it and say to myself, "You can do better; this is not who you were meant to be. Realize your potential and work hard at achieving it. You can do it! If not now, then never!"

This get-real moment was fueled with other horror stories from moms at the park. One lady confided in me that ever since the birth of her baby she had not been able to lose weight. I asked her how old her baby was, and she responded, "Oh, my son is five years old now."

How could this be? Five years had passed by with no weight loss. This could easily have been me, but I devised this program complete with a sound food plan and exercise routine to build lean muscle, melt off fat pounds, and add energy to my life, enabling me to look and feel my best! Now I am passing this wealth of information on to you so that you can also get the energy, stamina, and endurance you need to get through your day!

My advice is to take a "before" picture of yourself and ask, "What can be better? What would I like to change?" You can improve the way you look by following the Footsteps to Success principles, just as I did! I went from being a miserable, overweight mom to being crowned Ms. Bikini America and Ms. Muscle & Fitness after the birth of my second son by following a success blueprint! But it all starts in your mind, and this is what we will address in the next chapter.

My Story by Carolin Milder

I'm just like many of you reading this book. I'm a normal woman and a very busy mother of two cheeky little boys. I'm an extremely busy self-employed entrepreneur. And I love to work hard and focus on my business agendas and goals. I'm proud to say that I've created my life and have worked very hard to enjoy what I have. I'm blessed to be very happily married to my dream man. My husband and I truly enjoy experiencing the wonder of nature every day as my two boys grow up so quickly right before our eyes!

My husband and I work a lot so our family can enjoy a certain type of lifestyle. My roles and responsibilities with our company are never ending. On top of all that, I have to take care of my children, run a household, and look after the family dog. But I always schedule my workouts and eat right.

My professional career has been very interesting yet demanding. I have degrees in architecture and have been a trade representative in several industries, in addition to my long-time recruiting and headhunting business. Building the structure of my own headhunting company has taken a lot of time, patience, and hard work. But the great thing is that hard work pays off, and it has given my family and me much success.

But it even with hard work, it hasn't always been easy. After my second pregnancy, the global economic crisis hit us hard. I saw all of my blood, sweat, and tears just go down the drain. All of the dedication, time, and energy used to build my business had been for nothing. I was in complete shambles, and we almost lost everything!

Long story short, I was done. I was very close to suffering from depression due to the financial crash. I was home a lot with the kids, and so the emotional and mindless eating started to happen. I was suffering from confusion and felt so sad that I fed my emotions though food. I self-medicated with food, and lots of it!

At that time I weighed about 170 pounds, and I was miserable. My entire body was so sick, weak, and out of whack. I wasn't able to move properly, as I was so riddled with stress that my body was all locked up. I was so out of shape that when I climbed a flight of stairs, I ran out of breath! Also I had a hard time putting on my shoes, as I had a big belly in my way.

My self-confidence went right out the door! I didn't feel sexy or pretty at all. I didn't even like to have my own husband see me naked. I was just so lost, scared, and lonely. I had to do something fast, as it was only going to get worse if I didn't.

I look back at this now and realize that it was the most difficult time of our lives. My husband was permanently on the road to earn money for us. I was again left alone with my small children, fighting through the days to stay positive. My husband would make money on the road, but sadly enough it would just flow right out through the holes in our company! I'm sharing all of this with you so you can know that you are not alone in having personal hardships that affect your life. There are so shortcuts and no excuses, and if you want it badly enough, you will achieve your weight-loss goals!

Of course, this situation naturally impacted our marriage. I had to find a solution! I was so ready to make a positive change in my life. I was sad, tired, weak, and lonely. But I had to do something so I could get back in control of my life, my body, my business, and my marriage—and of course so I could be the best mom to my small children. So my search began! And as the saying goes, "When the student is ready, the teacher appears."

When my children went to sleep, my quest started. I searched online for diets, exercise, weight loss, and how to finally get in shape once and for all. And it happened—my "aha!" moment. I came across Jennifer Nicole Lee.

Who was this? She had such a similar history to mine, and she looked so amazing in the pictures—strong, sexy, powerful, success-ful, and desirable—that I was a loyal follower and the absolute JNL fan within a short time.

I had a new and definite goal, to become fit and successful just like JNL. I also wanted to have her goddess body, the stunning "superhero" charisma, and her contagious positive energy.

I know that the saying "ask and you shall receive" is true. I asked, and it happened! Thoughts become things! So now through my desire to get out of my own dark rut, I had found the solution and discovered that it is possible to have the life and body of your dreams. At that time, I had no idea what else would come to pass: our first book! You see, I'm here to tell you that I not only got in shape but also became more suc-cessful and fulfilled in my life.

After I got back on track, I began to really soak up the fitness information. I wanted to know and learn so much! I just had to find out how to crack my weight-loss code, how to train the right way for long-lasting weight-loss results. I look back now and celebrate having trained with the JNL Fusion exercise videos—and I can see just how they sparked my fitness fire!

Day after day I kept myself motivated to stay on my weight-loss journey by reading JNL's books, looking at her "before" and "after" photos, and also purchasing her other fitness products and programs. Of course, I read every page of her books and soaked up all the information like a sponge!

Losing weight, gaining sleek, sexy muscle tone, and getting in shape wasn't as hard as I thought it would be. I actually enjoyed it, and it was fun because I was following a successful fitness icon who *made* it fun, entertaining, and superengaging. JNL wasn't boring or too serious, which made me want to work out more. I actually looked forward to training with her and doing the workouts. Little by little my body got stronger, fitter, and better. I actually started to crave healthy food. I also began to feel more attractive and beautiful. This was a fantastic feeling. For once I loved the way I looked and felt. I wanted to take care of myself in order to fulfill my dream: to have a firm and enviable body that made me feel sexy and desirable, as well as lasting fitness and health. I was happy with myself, and I was happier with my husband and my kids; I just loved life so much. I was at my fullest potential and making the most of the once-horrible situation that the financial crisis had put me through.

I had found my passion. I finally got off my downward spiral and got onto my upward spiral. I became a certified personal-fitness trainer and trained myself for competitions as an elite IFBB Pro Figure fitness athlete. Then I decided to really go for it and sign up for my first fitness competition! I even went another step further by contacting JNL, as she was hosting one of her world-famous Fitness Model Factory one-day megaevents.

Jennifer was so excited about my story that she accepted me into their family and has since become my mentor. I have learned so much;

my business has grown, and now I'm proud to say that I am the number-one JNL Fusion master trainer of Germany.

I am incredibly grateful to JNL for this wonderful, life-changing, unique opportunity. It was my destiny to find these Footsteps to Success because now I can share them with you all and pay it forward!

At this point I would like to thank my wonderful mentor, Jennifer Nicole Lee:

Dear Jennifer,

I thank you from the bottom of my heart. You motivated me in the most difficult times in my life. You gave me direction when I was so lost. And you showed me the Footsteps to Success and helped me to achieve my goals. You believed in me when I didn't believe in myself.

As I followed in your successful footsteps, you gave me strength, discipline, and the necessary faith in myself. Without that belief, I never would have made it! You are forever my angel on earth! You have given me the greatest gift: faith! Faith to believe in myself and most importantly to never give up!

In true love, my sister,
Your Carolin

I still can't believe that I was once an overweight, depressed mom who had no clear vision of a promising future. And now, by following the Footsteps to Success, I am a professional fitness competitor. I still pinch myself because my body transformation was so evident that I have enjoyed a huge success in just my first professional competition season. In the spring of 2013, I even qualified for the German championship and was able to successfully place in the top five in the professional circuit.

To sum it all up, I am the complete Cinderella story. I went from the bottom straight to the top! I never gave up; I kept the faith, believed in myself, and continued following the Footsteps to Success. I lost almost eighty pounds for good, and now I enjoy being a fitness expert, coach, wellness consultant, and lifestyle expert in high demand—and now a published author. I was once a shy, overweight mom who hated her body, and now I love to fitness model and rock the camera! I also enjoy being a leader of the JNL Fusion workout method.

I'm so proud of my hard work and journey. I'm so glad that I finally got so eager to change my life that I found my mentor, Jennifer Nicole Lee, and have changed my life for good. My mission now is to pave the way for other women, moms, and out-of-shape people with these Footsteps to Success!

In closing I would like to encourage all mothers and women who are stressed and tired to end the madness and start working out and eating healthfully. You will become stronger for yourselves and for your families. Listen up, women: you have to make a decision now to work out, exercise, eat better, and take care of you. You must be strong for yourself and for your family and loved ones. And out of your physical strength, you will become mentally, emotionally, and spiritually strong. With this type of empowerment, you will start to really love the life you're living!

Jennifer and I have learned from our own weight-loss success what to do and what not to do, so we invite you to take this new, exciting fitness journey with us. We know the exact Footsteps to Success that will lead you straight to the goals you deserve. We know you can do it because we've done it ourselves. Read this entire book and live by it. Not only will you get your physical body in order but you will start to experience confidence and success in all areas of your life.

We believe in *you*!

Strong is the new skinny!

JNL and CM

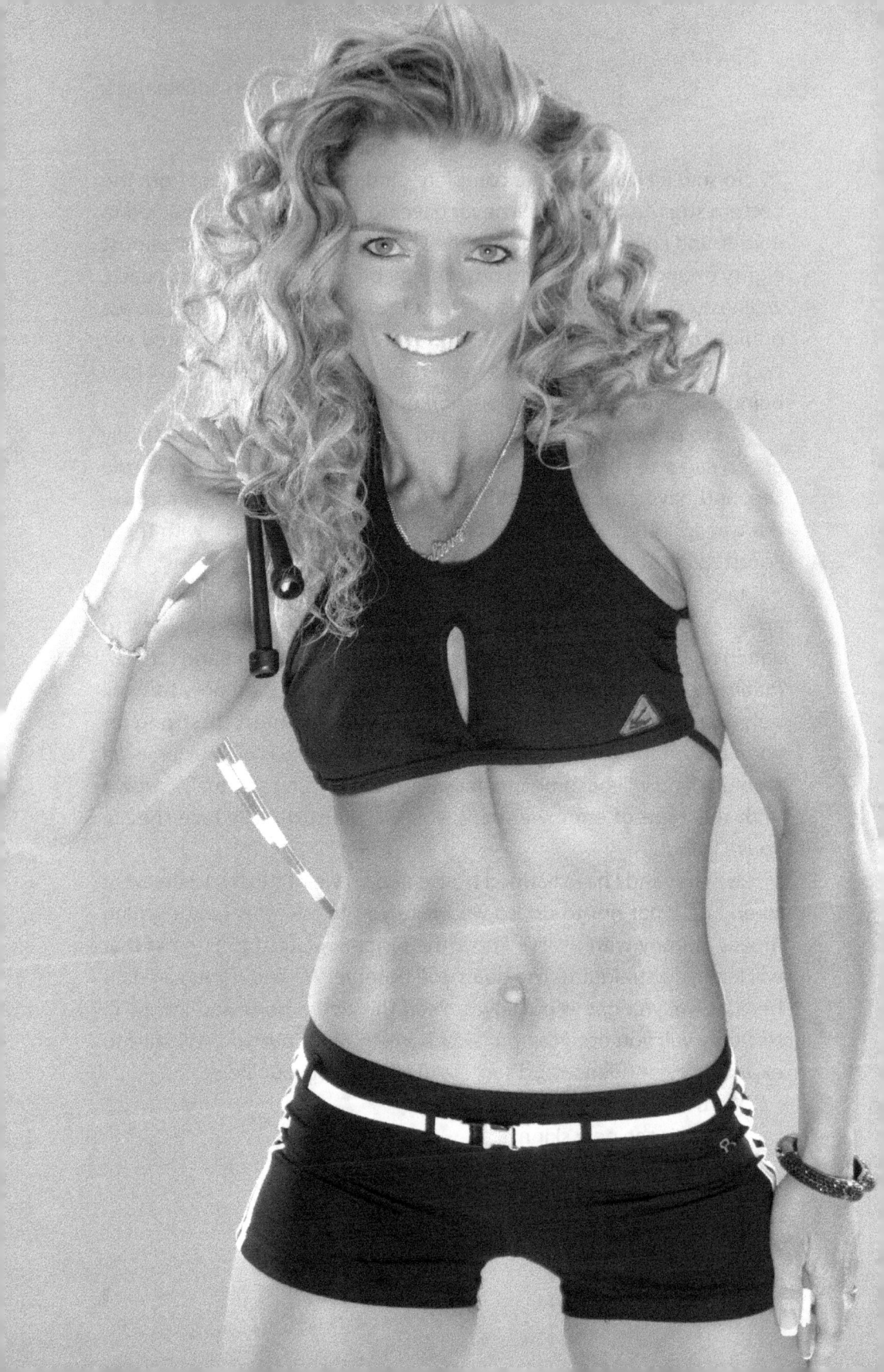

CHAPTER 2

Why Fad Diets Are Dangerous, Don't Work, and Cause Harm

It's unfortunate to say that we have all gone on a fad diet. We have all been victims lured into following these quick-fix gimmicks. They lead to rapid weight loss, which then turns back into diet relapse with, sadly enough, the pounds back on us. Sometimes we even gain more weight back because we've damaged our metabolism. It has happened to the best of us, from Oprah Winfrey to Princess Diana to some of the biggest names in the entertainment industry—and yes, to you and to us.

First of all, fad quick-fix diets are extremely dangerous for many reasons. During one of these diets, your body is always living with a constant shortage of energy. You are left irritable, tired, and fatigued. Many times these diets are deficient in the nutrients that your body needs to function properly, which can lead to hair loss, low energy, and lack of drive. You then yo-yo up and down. You lose weight; then you gain the weight back. It's a vicious cycle.

These fad diets are everywhere you look! Just take a glimpse at your local magazine rack, and you'll find many of them being advertised in attractive, glossy ads. We know this all too well because we were once in this vicious cycle.

You know the old saying "it's too good to be true"? Well, most people instinctively know that these fad diets don't work, but the "before" and "after" photos, the promises made, and the attractive marketing can fool even the best of us! And the sad thing is that these quick-fix fad diets are very dangerous for many reasons.

What Exactly Happens during a Diet?
Most diets are based on a reduction of nutritional value; for example, calorie intake is reduced, and the body is forced to draw on its own reserves.

As a side effect, metabolism switches to "emergency mode" because it thinks you're starving. Thus, your metabolism slows down to hold onto the fat, energy, and calories in your body. This is exactly what we don't want. We don't want a broken-down or burned-out metabolism because we will have a very difficult time shedding the weight safely and with long-term results.

Simply put, on a quick-fix diet, your metabolism is steadily getting slower and burning fewer calories; in other words it's storing fuel, which ends up being fat.

It's sad to say that many women—and men—have dealt with this problem, especially fitness and fashion models. They are forced to eat less and exercise more to be thinner. Thus, their metabolism slows down. But it's a vicious cycle. They need to keep doing more and more cardio training so that they can maintain their weight.

Overtraining and undereating are other forms of an unhealthy lifestyle. But many of us fall into this dangerous trap. We want instant results, so we go to extreme measures to achieve weight loss that normally takes two months. We want the results of two months in two weeks. But again, these results are temporary. We lose the weight initially, but then we gain it back, plus some more! We also end up with a damaged metabolism, which causes us to hold on to the fat.

When we go into this vicious cycle of overtraining and undereating, we actually burn our muscles and not fat. This is exactly what we don't want, because our muscles are our golden ticket to lifelong weight loss, energy, endurance, and stamina. Our muscles are our fountain of youth, giving us athletic performance. We must protect them, and not burn them out.

It has been proven that the more muscle mass someone has, the higher her metabolism. Our goal is to have a very efficient metabolism so we burn off calories easily and more quickly. To put it in simple terms, the more muscle mass you have, the more calories and fat you will naturally burn, so in turn you can eat more calories without gaining weight as quickly as others. Therefore your goal should be to build lean, athletic muscle mass and to lose fat.

Weight Loss Versus Inch Loss

We must also change our mindset from weight loss to inch loss. Because muscle weighs more than fat, you may not lose many pounds, but you will lose fat inches. So when you gain muscle and lose fat, you will actually shrink, getting smaller, tighter, and more toned. You will not bulk up and get big. You will replace the fat with lean muscle mass, reshaping your body. So again, let us repeat: it is not primarily about the weight loss but about gaining muscle and losing fat.

Here's a great tip: in addition to your scale, also track your progress by measuring your body with a measuring tape. With a tape measure, you will be able to see where you are losing the fat and the inches. This is a great way to track and celebrate your progress.

How to Stop Yo-Yoing

We have all been there, done that—we start our crash diet and experience the worst days of our lives. We eat little to nothing and exercise obsessively. We then find ourselves so weak, frail, and sometimes dizzy that we can't even stand up and walk. We are also so hungry that we would eat the paint off the walls! And then we give in and binge like crazy, eating everything in sight. And then we go right back to starving ourselves. It's a very vicious, unhealthy cycle.

Yes, the pounds might start to fall off, and at first we are overjoyed! Of course, we think this will go on forever and that we're on the right track. Finally we've reached our goal and our favorite dress fits again. But then the yo-yo effect happens, and we binge, overeat, and gain the weight right back!

This weight gain happens because we have damaged our metabolism, and no matter the diet or exercise we do, our body holds onto the fat and won't let it go. Again, our body thinks it's starving, so it hoards the fat.

The only solution to this dilemma is to provide our body with everything it needs to function properly. But how is this possible if we want to lose weight? This is where the Footsteps to Success are very important.

I (Carolin) know this vicious yo-yo dieting cycle all too well. In Germany we call her "JoJo," and I dealt with her before my pregnancies. I was always ready to start the next diet to break through and end this vicious cycle of weight loss and weight gain. However, it was always in vain. I always had three clothing sizes in my closet: 6, 8, and 10. And after the birth of my children, I was even starting to wear sizes 12 to 14!

Seeing these huge sizes and wearing these big clothes was just way too much of a nightmare for me. I had to change something and quick! I knew the Footsteps to Success were out there, and I got on a mission to find them. I just knew it because I saw all the superfit women and moms out there with endless energy and athletic muscle tone.

I was overjoyed when I started to see my own fat suit melt off, revealing the strong, fit me that was locked inside. The amazing thing was that I had lost almost eighty pounds. But what I was most excited about what that the vicious cycle of yo-yoing had finally been broken, and I was now living a fit and healthy lifestyle without hunger and cravings.

With this success, I made the decision to enter into a professional fitness competition. Competing as a fitness athlete makes balancing diet and exercise a tad more difficult, as you really need to dial in your physique. I lowered my body-fat percentage by a further 8 percent and lost another seventeen pounds. I was fully ripped, not an ounce of fat with pure, strong, tight, and toned muscle.

This precontest period is extremely hard. You must follow a very strict diet and pretty much give up everything you like to eat for a certain period of time, which is hard even though I love to compete because it challenges me to be my best.

But what came to me after this hard diet were the most horrible cravings I have ever experienced. They were so dramatic that I almost didn't come to grips with them. I read and researched an incredible amount about the time *after* the competition season and learned that this time is the most difficult stage because the body is forced to use up all its supplies for several months. In this situation, the yo-yo effect is much worse than in an average diet! Within two weeks I gained almost ten pounds. I felt so frustrated and helpless. I now know that I should have strictly adhered to a so-called building diet to get my metabolism back on track and to get my body back to a more natural, everyday diet, and this extreme weight gain would not have happened.

In closing, the good news is that when you follow a balanced, nutritious food plan along with a great workout program, you will enjoy permanent weight loss without suffering from the extreme yo-yoing nightmare.

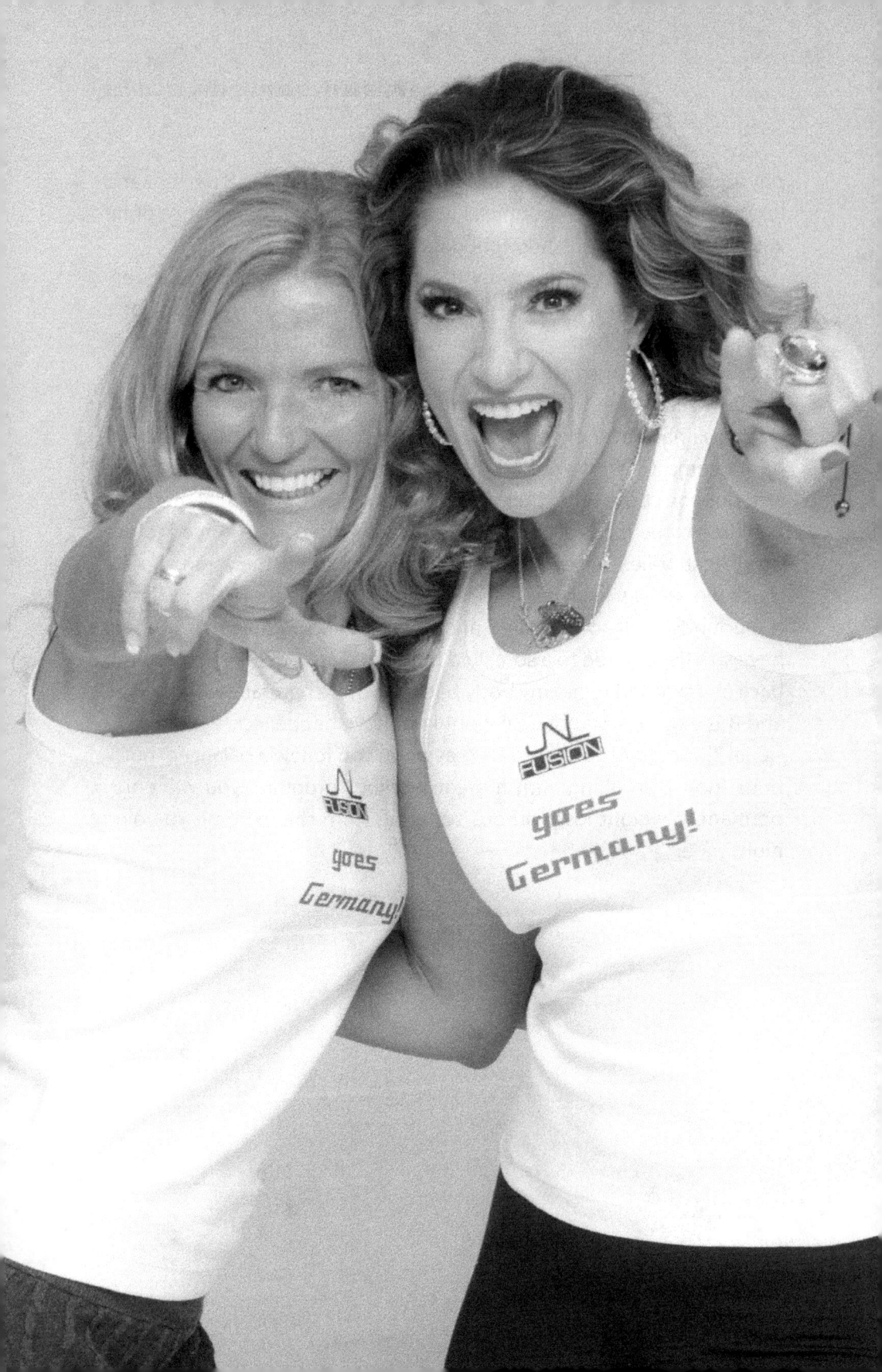

CHAPTER 3

Fitness Is Not a One-Time Dreaded Event but a Lifelong Journey to Be Enjoyed

In this chapter we are going to talk about finally moving away from fad diets and into living a fit, healthy, and balanced lifestyle.

It may sound strange, but if you want to lose weight permanently and enjoy having a slim, sexy, and strong body then you have to eat! Yes, you read this correctly! You have to eat the right food. In order to burn fat, you have to build sleek and sexy muscle tone. In order to build muscle tone, you must "feed" your muscle high-quality sources of lean protein. So again, starving yourself on a fad diet does more harm than good, as it slows down your metabolism and puts your body into starvation mode, which causes your body to hold on to the fat.

The plain and simple truth is that your body needs energy to burn off energy, so you must eat, and eat well. It's just like a car that needs gasoline in order to run. We cannot expect our bodies to function at a top performance level when we give them insufficient energy. But that's exactly what so many of us have done to our own bodies. We need foods high in nutritional value for them to run at an optimal level, but instead we eat "empty" calories that provide no nutritional value, such as sugary junk food, fatty fast food, or processed foods high in preservatives.

The successful way to feed our bodies with the right fuel, lose body fat, and build lean, strong muscles is the "fit and healthy" lifestyle. But does this mean that we are going to eat diet foods or "eat like a rabbit," eating little to nothing?

Absolutely not!

Our body needs a balanced diet full of whole-grain carbs, fibrous carbs, lean sources of high-quality protein, and heart-healthy fats.

There are many diets out there that are very strict and focus on the omission of either carbs, protein, or fats, thus making them unbalanced. For example the Paleo diet is based on a high-protein and high-fat intake, while carbohydrates are often omitted. Low-fat diets, on the other hand, are low in heart-healthy fats your body needs, such as omega-3 and -6. The list goes on and on.

However, none of these diets are balanced.

We are here to bust the diet myths and show you the footsteps to a successful diet. There are no "diet cards," no "phases," no "steps" or "for two weeks do this and for two weeks do that" stages. We're going to keep it simple, short, and sweet with good, solid, proven information that will be transformed into power in your life.

Many people think that carbs will make you fat. The truth is that we need whole-grain carbs for our bodies to function properly and as part of a balanced diet. The fact is that our bodies need carbohydrates for energy. But we must be clear about the *type* of carbs we need to eat. Go for whole-grain carbs such as oatmeal, brown rice, quinoa, barley, and whole-wheat breads and pastas. Stay away from the white breads, rice, and pastas.

While we're on the subject of carbs, a lot of the latest and most popular diets instruct you to cut out fruit. Fruit in the Footsteps to Success program is a powerful superfood that is essential. How could the top fitness experts tell you not to eat fruit for two weeks? How misleading! As a specialist in sports nutrition, I (Jennifer) would never ask you to do something so ridiculous, harmful, and unsafe. Of course, if you don't eat sweets or have alcohol the first two weeks of any diet, you will lose weight. That isn't rocket science, and you don't need to be a doctor to know that. In this lifestyle program you will be shown not only how to get the number on the scale down but how to keep it down forever while you gain strength and get the energy in your body up! You will also improve the look and feel of your body inside and out.

In chapter 6, we will talk more about the "right" foods, how much to eat, what are the best times to eat, and of course, lots of delicious, mouthwatering recipes.

And the fantastic thing is that you'll have no more cravings—and even if you do, you'll know how to handle them, and you will be able to keep your dream figure long term!

The great news is that achieving your superfit, healthy body is still much easier than you think! We are here to show you how to work along with your amazing body by feeding it highly nutritious meals, instead of working against it by starving yourself on a fad diet.

The Importance of Macronutrients
The balance of macronutrients (carbs, fat, and protein) is very important. And contrary to popular opinion, all of these body-building materials are healthy and essential to a high-performance, healthy, and attractive body.

Many popular diet approaches recommend greatly reducing or even banning fat or carbohydrates, but in the long term this is not healthy, and it is certainly not a balanced diet, not to mention that it is very difficult to sustain. The trick is to give the body everything it needs in order to increase fat burning to the highest level.

Let's look at macronutrients individually to see how each is important.

Carbohydrates
Carbs are a vital source of energy; they give us strength and are our fuel. Carbs are found in fruit, pasta, rice, grains, and sugar. Each gram of carbohydrates contains four calories. In the body, carbohydrates

are turned into glucose, a specific type of sugar, before they reach our bloodstream.

The key to understanding which carbohydrates are healthy and which are not is their rate of degradation, which regulates blood-sugar levels. This speed is called the "glycemic index." Blood-sugar levels in turn are responsible for the secretion of the hormone insulin. A rapid rate of carbohydrate degradation results in a high insulin release. Due to this rapid degradation of glucose in the blood, fatigue and cravings are triggered more rapidly, giving a clear signal to the body to gain fat.

So-called "simple" carbohydrates have a very fast rate of degradation. That's one of the reasons why we should avoid table sugar and white flour. Choose instead brown rice, whole-wheat pasta, whole-grain bread, couscous, and buckwheat as side dishes. These healthy "complex" carbohydrates keep your blood sugar stable so that your cravings become a thing of the past.

All vegetables and fruits also contain natural carbohydrates, but you can eat as much as you like of them until you are fully satisfied—with the exception of potatoes, peas, carrots, and sweet potatoes. Treat these starchy vegetables like you would brown rice, whole grains, and whole-wheat bread—just a small portion will suffice. The bulk of your meal should consist of vegetables and a lean protein source.

Protein
Protein is the most important but most neglected macronutrient. It is required not only for muscle maintenance but also to build muscle. Amino acids are the smallest component of proteins, which are used for the repair and regeneration of our body's cells. You should incorporate a lean source of protein into every meal, for example, protein powder, chicken, turkey, skim cottage cheese, lean beef, fish, or eggs.

Fat
Fat is not your enemy! It is your friend, and believe it or not, it helps in the process of weight loss. Burning fat requires eating fat—but the

healthy kind, such as nuts, seeds, high-quality extra-virgin olive oil, avocado, coconut oil, and fish oils.

Fat should make up about 25 to 30 percent of your daily calories. So have no fear of a handful of almonds, two tablespoons of peanut butter, or an avocado as a snack. These are all rich in fat and do contain calories, but the healthy fats boost your metabolism and make you burn fat.

Water

One of the biggest obstacles to weight loss is dehydration. Most people do not drink enough water; the result is that they get headaches, feel weak, and wonder why they are so limp and tired.

This is a classic case of dehydration! The body shuts down its engines and burns less fuel so that its systems do not "burn out" in the truest sense of the word.

Do you drink only when you're thirsty? Then you are already dehydrated! A good rule of thumb is to drink one cup of water at least eight times per day, equivalent to about two to three liters. That is the minimum; more is better in this case. Water is essential to your body, flushing out the blood vessels, cleaning the body and helping it make repairs, renewing cells, and stimulating fat burning. Drink yourself slim with water!

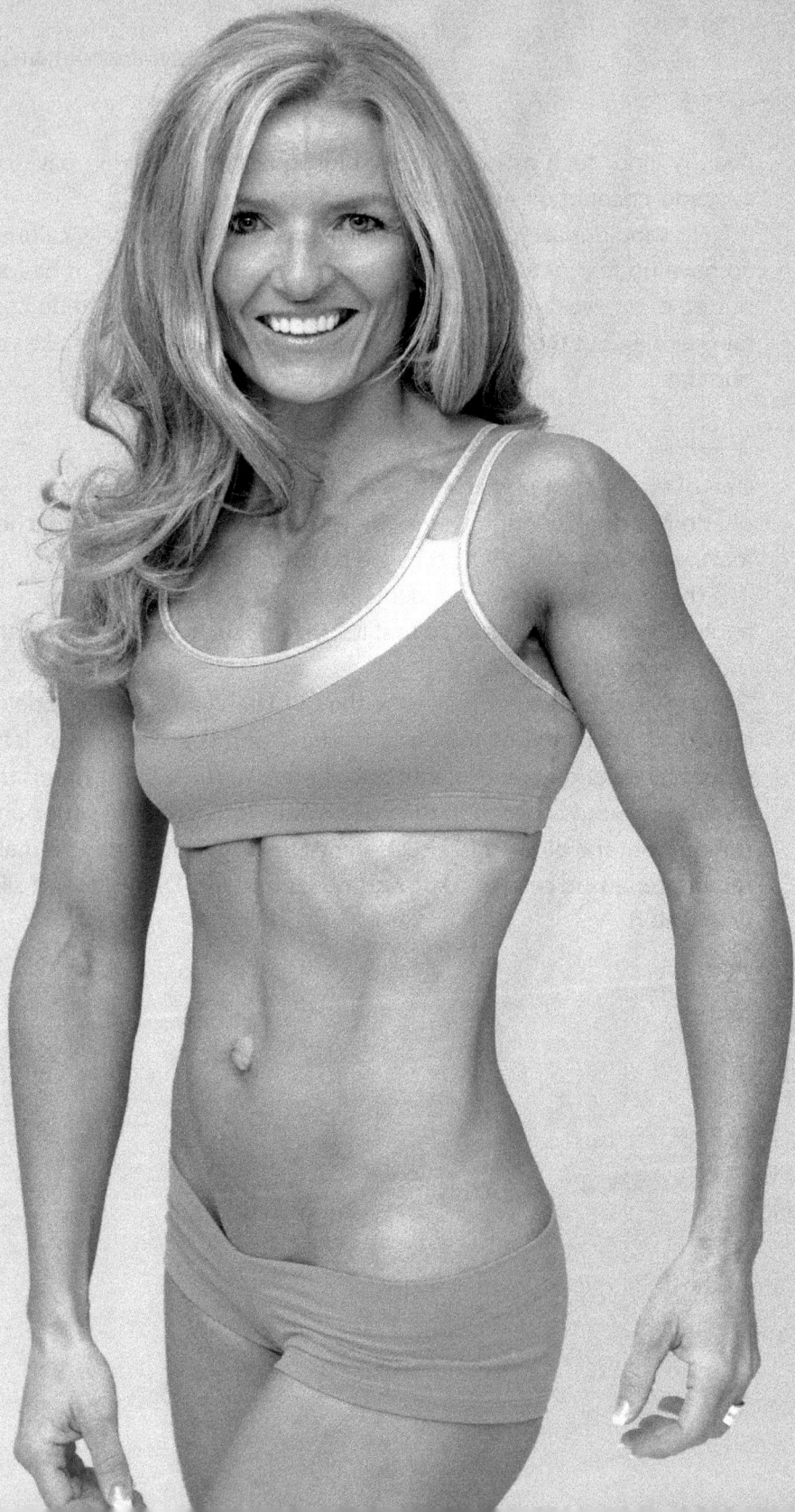

CHAPTER 4

Your Mind Is Your Strongest Muscle and Your Brain Is Your Body's Engine

Start exercising with the most important workout—the workout from your neck up!
—Jennifer Nicole Lee

One of the most important aspects to address before starting a complete transformational health program is preparing yourself for the miracles that are going to come your way. As a life coach, I (Jennifer) spend an immense amount of time with my personal clients, getting them ready for the amazing journey ahead of them. I have found, through my experience, that the key to achieving magical results is to make sure my clients are mentally prepared and committed to making these improvements in their lives.

You see, merely being interested in a thing is a wholly different mindset than being committed to it. In order for you to create positive transformations, you must be committed to making the necessary changes in your life that will yield success. How do you get prepared? By making sure you are fully focused, dedicated, and ready to take on your brand-new life. How do you get to this point? I like to take my personal clients through an exercise I call the Pre–Footsteps to Success Consultation.

In this exercise, take some quiet time to carefully consider your past and present states. Ask yourself these empowering questions.

Pre–Footsteps to Success Consultation
1. If I continue with my current lifestyle, where will I be in one year? Two years? Five years? Ten years?
2. Is what I am doing currently working for me or against me?
3. Am I living my life to its utmost potential?
4. If I don't make the necessary changes in my life, starting today, where will my life end up?
5. Am I totally, fully happy with my life now?
6. Am I ready to prove to myself, my family, and the world just how amazing I am?
7. Do I accept that, in order to become an example of personal excellence, I must go above and beyond my own expectations and also the expectations of others?
8. Up until now, have I really amazed myself and those close to me with my own abilities?
9. Do I understand that to be a winner, I must learn from other winners?
10. Do I fully comprehend that during my journey to become my best, there will be times of frustration and growing pains through which I must persevere in order to achieve my desired results?

While following the Footsteps to Success program, you'll experience a new level of excitement thanks to your changed lifestyle and fitness freedom. You will be blessed with the energy that comes from health, healing, and happiness.

But you may also experience down times, difficulties, and challenges. Be steadfast! Stay focused on your goals. Remember, keeping your eye on the prize is essential to your victory. Many people will try to distract you and deter you. Revisit your Footsteps to Success principles—and rededicate yourself to your goals.

At times, you may feel that you are moving too slowly toward your desired outcome. You may ask yourself, "Why haven't I lost weight yet? Why isn't this working faster? Why don't I have the body of my dreams by now?" When these negative feelings boil up, remind yourself that success doesn't happen overnight. Striving for personal excellence in all areas of your life takes patience and persistence. If you have to undo years of inward and outward resistance and negative conditioning, it will take more time.

Just sit back, relax, take a big, deep breath in, and then exhale. You are about to embark on one of the most magical and miraculous times of your life. Just know that you will reach your goals if you stick to the principles outlined in this book. Like my own transformation, it won't happen overnight—but it will happen! Because I refused to give up or give in, I've been given the gift to motivate you to create your dream life. I'm proud to pass the torch of wisdom to you so that you, too, can succeed in all areas of your life—through health, healing, and happiness.

If you're getting results but you hit a plateau, don't let it sap your motivation. It's only natural to hit plateaus. Think of it as a "rest area" to ramp up for the amazing benefits to come. It's like pulling into a rest stop on a long road trip and taking a pause to refuel and get reorganized for the remainder of your journey. Don't waste your time getting frustrated. Plateaus happen to everyone, in every aspect of life—especially when you're learning something new. Success comes in waves, like the ocean. So, when a wave of success is on its way out, use that down time to strategize and prepare for your continued progress.

As anyone who has ever learned to play a new sport or musical instrument, or gone to college to learn a new trade, will tell you, there is always a learning curve, as well as plateaus along the way. It's how we handle this experience that separates the losers from the winners. A winner is a loser who picks herself up that one last time and continues on. So keep plugging along. This is when you must be committed to your success, not just interested in it.

Remember, your actions are your results and then ultimately become your life!

Health starts in the mind and then flows to the body.
—Jennifer Nicole Lee

Cleaning Your Mental House

Before you even start a new healthy-lifestyle program, you must "clean your mental house" and prepare your mind. As a life coach and mentor, I'm going to help you prep both the mind and body for the fantastic health advances that lie ahead. You must be 100 percent committed to making healthy progress in order to see and keep results!

Although it may be hard to be believe, sometimes we sabotage our own success because we are not mentally ready or committed to sticking to our wonderful lifestyle improvements. You must create your results before they occur and prepare yourself for boundless energy and confidence. In order to lose unwanted fat pounds, you must start with your mind!

A close friend of mine sabotaged her weight-loss potential by saying to herself, "Why lose weight? My skin will only be flabby if I lose the amount of weight I want." She had already set herself up for failure by predetermining that she wasn't going to lose weight.

Another client of mine once claimed that she wanted to lose weight but was afraid of all the remarks from those close to her, and how it might affect her family. I told her that she would only be adding quality to her life, not taking away from it—and that these healthy new changes would actually be helping her family as well. What about the added health risks of heart disease and diabetes, not to mention the added pressure on joints from additional weight? In addition, the other side to this fear was rooted in the constant idea that she would never be able to lose weight.

These are examples of people riding the fence, not knowing what side to get off on. Make a decision to improve your life by being healthy, because your mind and body will thank you.

Preparing Yourself Mentally to Lose Weight

Start by asking yourself, "Do I have a healthy mind or a mind that will thwart my efforts? Am I my own best friend or my worst enemy?"

If you answered yes to the latter, we first need to clean your mental house!

Here are our top seven Footsteps to Success strategies for giving yourself the right mental attitude that will allow you to start improving your life.

1. Have a crystal-clear vision of what you want to achieve.
We've heard it so many times. Clients come to us and cry, "I'm sick and tired of being overweight! I have no energy, and I'm tired all the time."

This will not help you! We all know what we want to move away from. But what do we want to move toward? We're referring to the fact that you must realize where your main focus needs to be in order for you to achieve weight-loss success from now on. Since we have all taken a "before" picture of ourselves, we need to now have an "after" image of what we want.

Envision what you want to achieve. See the new you, and imagine what it would feel like to *be* that new you! Take out your journal and write down what you want to achieve, what you want to move toward, and how you are going to do it. Picture yourself with limitless energy, able to handle your daily tasks and/or your job, all the while still having enough steam leftover for your children and your personal life. How will it feel to put on a swimsuit and feel great about what you see in the mirror?

Imagine weighing yourself and loving the number you see! You will start to relish the afterburn of your morning workouts! You have to know and understand what you are moving toward and say good-bye to what you are moving away from to be able to have fitness success and maintain it.

2. Clean out your mental house.
Stop putting yourself down! That unfriendly little voice inside your head needs to be silenced now and forever. That supercritical, opinionated alter ego of yours needs to know who the boss is. You are! So what if you gained five pounds on the family vacation cruise? That does not make you a "fat pig." Rather than beating yourself up by complaining, compliment yourself by saying something like "Yeah, I did have that chocolate-chip cookie for dessert. But I didn't have three of them like I would have done before."

You need to learn to stay focused on your objective and stay positive. Don't let the negativity get you down or blur the vision you have of your destination. Stop whining, and take more control over your actions and your life. Stop playing the victim. It doesn't help you or others around you.

3. Treat yourself with respect.

Respect yourself. It's that simple, but we don't do it. If you had a best friend whom you loved with all your might, would you give her a fat-laden, artery-clogging cheeseburger with fries or a crisp and fresh garden salad topped with grilled chicken? Yes, you would give her the salad. But why don't you do this for yourself? Most likely because the psychology behind your actions does not allow you to treat yourself with the respect and consideration you have for those you love. You are self-sacrificing, always giving to others and not yourself.

Think about this: your mind and body are temples, and you need to treat them as such. Why would you put something dirty and of no value in a sacred and special place?

Well, of course you wouldn't. So start respecting yourself and treating yourself right. You deserve better than processed fast food with little to no healthy nutrient content. Also, you deserve to chisel out at least fifty minutes every other day for a weight-training session with a touch of cardio at the end. Remember, you are the most important person in your life. If you can't help yourself, then how can you help others? It all begins with you!

4. Be creative.

What do we mean by this? We don't mean you need to be an artist or a philosophical thinker. But we are in this life for the long run. Being healthy is a process, a journey, not a one-time event. Fitness and health are going to be your new lifestyle. Therefore, you need to find the things that make this journey fun—the sport that gives you energy and new foods and recipes to try so that you have some variety and aren't pursuing the same boring routine day after day.

Ask yourself, "What are my favorite foods and the exercises I love to do most?" If you answered Italian food, then buy a low-fat, low-carb Italian cookbook and learn how to remake your old favorites! And if you love to play tennis, join a tennis club or hire an instructor who will help you strengthen your backhand or give you a better edge on your game. If you love nachos, be creative and reinvent the recipe using low-fat ingredients rather than the real stuff.

You're the most important person in your life. Do things you enjoy that make you feel special, like a nice bath with candlelight in the evening when the kids are asleep, or a walk in the sunlight. Just open your mind to new and different tools, and use them as a bag of tricks that will help you fight the war on fat. By being creative, you will make it fun, refreshing, and interesting. There will never be a dull moment in your new, healthy life.

5. Put fitness first.
Well, not exactly first, but make it a top priority. Exercise should be a rock in your life. If your car breaks down, exercise. If you get a job promotion, exercise. If your husband leaves you, exercise. No matter what happens—stick to your routine!

Of course, we all will have bad days and get off of our healthy food plans—but refocus yourself, look at your compass, and get back on track! And prepare to be tempted. This strategy of "thinking five steps ahead" will allow you to win at the game of fat loss. If you know that you have to attend your family's barbeque dinner with nonstop servings of hot dogs, potato salad, and sugary desserts, be smart and execute your fitness plan: munch on a crispy apple before the barbecue. This will fill you up, cutting the edge off any uncontrollable hunger pains that might set in while you're there. Then opt for the grilled chicken breast with no bun, a side salad, and an ear of corn with no butter. You'll be putting fitness first, and you'll still be able to enjoy your family's social activities without sabotaging your fitness goals.

6. Set yourself up for success.
Put health on the shelf and the gym bag in the car. Stock your fridge and pantry with the latest guilt-free snacks and treats. Low-carb and low-fat foods are tasting better and better. Try something new today. Have your gym bag ready to go in the car for a pre- or postworkday workout. Throw in a towel and a change of clothes, and you'll have no excuse to skip the gym.

Everywhere you go and no matter where you are, your healthy habits will follow you. Therefore it will be almost impossible to not stick to your plan and reach your goals. Buy used exercise DVDs for little to nothing online and have them ready to go in your family room. Have your running shoes right by the bed so all you have to do is roll out of the sack and into your morning run!

7. Compel and coerce through pain.

Yes, pain *can* be your friend! Use it to your advantage as a tool to get you motivated to make a positive change in your life. We created our success through constantly reminding ourselves of what we looked like before, and of the pain we experienced when we were at our heaviest.

Get some leverage on yourself. First, it is absolutely necessary for you to take a "before" picture of yourself. Second, it would be best if you took this "before" picture and put it somewhere you can occasionally see it when you need to feel the "pain" and frustration associated with that picture to get you motivated. When you feel your motivation and desire weakening, glance at the picture and remind yourself of the despair you felt when you were at your unhealthiest. To make yourself take action, you have to be at the threshold of pain, looking directly at it. This is where your power and supremacy over your future decisions will come from.

Pain will be your friend because you will learn how to manipulate it and use it to your advantage. The pain that we revisited often was surrounded by our overweight "before" photos. We deliberately glanced at our "before" images to use them as our pain, and that coerced us into taking positive action.

This pain was the vital vehicle that propelled us into fast-forward mode, making sure we never pushed the rewind button. We used the pain of feeling overweight and frumpy and not being able to wear the beautiful clothes we wanted to as a therapeutic medium to move toward our goals. These were all the methods that led to our weight-loss achievements.

Again, please use these techniques to stay on the right path. When you look at your "before" picture...

- Remember how you felt carrying all that extra weight around.
- Remember how you were treated differently when you were heavier.
- Remember the confidence you started to experience when you felt stronger.
- Compare your old lifestyle with your new, improved one and how great it feels to live a healthy, fit, and strong lifestyle.

And as we speak from experience, we can't say it enough: it is necessary to stop playing the victim and start making those improvements in your life *now* to become victorious!

Remember, your mind is the strongest muscle in your body. So once you make the decision to control it, you will achieve your goals. Your mind has the power to either be your worst enemy or your best positive, supportive friend.

Get your "before" photo and hang it up everywhere. Post it in your bathroom, bedroom, in the kitchen. Seeing your "before" photo will be the driving catalyst to help you to continue on your positive journey and to follow your Footsteps to Success.

8. Use superpositive affirmations.

While sometimes there is nothing more powerful than a decision from the depths of your pain, a positive outlook is just as necessary to achieving success. Keep positive and only think good, loving thoughts about yourself, and you will enjoy your journey to the new, fit you!

Remember this very important rule in life: the past does not equal the future. We are the result of our past negative experiences. So how can we create the future we want when we're always looking into the rearview mirror at our past? When we have had a negative experience, we store it in our brains as a just that, and all other similar experiences are automatically perceived from the outset as negative.

Now transfer this idea to the subject of weight loss. How many diets have you already tried, and what were your results? Have you ever achieved your dream body? If so, what torments and limitations did you have to endure to do so? The usual madness of diets is that we strictly adhere to the diet plan until we finally reach our destination on the scale, but a few weeks later, the whole circus was in vain because we've gained the same weight back if not more! Then come a few weeks of frustration, and that's the start of the next catastrophic diet. And the cycle begins again!

So this time, we are going to "flush" all the negativity and embrace the new, positive future of our weight loss by following the Footsteps to Success in order to achieve our fitness goals.

You have to get these negative experiences out of your head. You cannot be afraid of the next failure, because there is no longer any failure. You *will* be able to change your lifestyle and take care of yourself, your body, and the well-being and health of your family.

This is how you begin to reprogram all your negative beliefs. This technique works on all levels, but let's start with your great figure, and then you can apply your knowledge to other life situations.

Affirmations are simple techniques that help you create new thoughts. These are phrases that describe your ideal state. You can either read these silently to yourself or repeat them out loud. Here are some examples for you:

- I am fit and healthy.
- I am strong and sexy.
- I reach my goals and am always brave.
- Strong is the new skinny.
- I believe in myself.
- I'm doing what is right and important for me.
- I live my dream life and am always positive and open.
- Any difficult situation makes me grow and become stronger.
- I look forward to each new day.
- My day is fantastic, and I enjoy my life.
- I love healthy eating and feeling good in my body.

Affirmations are always positive because we want your thoughts to become positive and powerful.

Jennifer Nicole Lee has absolutely perfected this technique with her own fashion brand, JNL Clothing, which features strong affirmations. You can wear your favorite shirts each day and remind yourself of what you stand for and what goals you have. Order today at www.JNLClothing.com.

9. Believe in yourself.
Out of all these mental-preparation techniques, the most important is your own belief in yourself. Sometimes believing in yourself is hard to do. Sometimes the people around you will try to persuade you to not believe in yourself. This is when your inner champion must come out and believe in you even when others don't.

In these situations it may be difficult to stay on track from time to time. Never give up! Don't let challenges and negative people prevent you from reaching your dreams and goals. These are *your* dreams, *your* goals, and *you* will create them! It's your life, and you've earned the right to live it the way you want to and to feel good in your body as well.

And don't forget to reward yourself for reaching your goals each step of the way—for example, with a nice summer dress when you've lost a size, or a pampering afternoon at the spa with a massage.

Learn to love you—no matter what your body looks like at this moment! If you love yourself, you'll look and take care of yourself by doing the right things in order to create your dream body.

Love for your body and your soul starts in your mind. Make it a goal to tell yourself every day how wonderful you are and that you're doing a great job. When I (Carolyn) weighed almost two hundred pounds, I hated my body and the fact that I had allowed myself to look like this! I refused to buy new clothes or look in the mirror. I was wearing my old, not-very-nice-looking pregnancy clothes. Some days I didn't care what I ate, how I looked, or how I felt. Other days I ate almost nothing in an effort to finally lose weight and to punish myself for the situation I was stuck in. And of course, after a few days I was back at the other end of the spectrum with intense cravings, eating everything I could get my hands on. I bathed in self-pity and hate.

My thoughts were way more negative than they should have been due just to having a difficult time with my business. I was living a nightmare, and I wanted to wake up from it.

However, I had the good fortune to find a very good friend and mentor who taught me that the beginning is always love of self! It's hard to believe at first, and it's hard to start acting on, but it's the truth. When I finally started to love, appreciate, and accept the way I was, that was the beginning of change. I started enjoying seeing myself in the mirror again, even before I had my ideal figure—I was finally on the right track, and that alone was great!

You can reach all your goals if you love and accept yourself, which is the start to believing in yourself.

10. Learn something new every day.
If you keep doing the same things, you'll keep getting the same results. This saying has motivated us again and again to learn new things so we can become better every day and keep moving forward step by step toward our goals and desires.

Do you want different results than in the past? This means you have to do things differently—much differently from what you've done so far based on what you already know.

The nice thing is that there are always people who have taken a similar path ahead of you, and you can learn from them how it works and in what direction you need to go.

On the way to your dream figure and a happy and healthy life, we want to show you everything you need to know to find your direction, because it's not as difficult as you may think. You've already learned a lot from this book, and you will continue to increase your knowledge as you read on.

The important thing is, however, not only to read and to know but also to *apply* these new techniques and practices in your everyday life. You can even improve upon them by your own application, because every person has her own rhythm in family and professional life.

Learning a new way of life is like learning a foreign language. At first it's hard and comes with difficulty, but if you keep going, hour after hour, week after week, year after year, you get better until you finally speak the language without even thinking about it, and you can talk with other people who are fluent.

Or let's take it to an even more basic level. What was it like in the first grade when you learned to read and write? At first it was difficult, but year after year you got better, and now you probably can't even imagine that you ever could not read or write.

Integrating a new way of life doesn't happen overnight. Rather, every day it happens a bit more. Each week in this program will instill something new in your life, something that will eventually feel completely normal, just like reading and writing.

Keep it simple! Make it a goal to incorporate these small, yet powerful, changes into your life. The new healthy habits will end up sticking and giving you the results you deserve.

How to Replace Old, Unhealthy Habits with New, Healthy Habits

Humans exist in a state of habit. Everything we do every day—how we dress, what we eat, and how we conduct ourselves and educate our children—is part of our habits. These habits shape us so much, and it's hard to break them. We notice this especially if we try to make a change! The first day it works, but the second is already difficult, and on the third day we fall back into old habits.

What are your habits? How you start your day? What do you have for breakfast? What do you give your kids as a snack in their lunch boxes? How do you decide what to wear? All these are your habits and make you into what you are at this moment.

In order to improve ourselves and our results significantly, we need to change our daily habits—and be deliberate about it. Studies have proven that the human brain requires thirty days to integrate something new like a habit. Only after these thirty days is a habit established in our minds as a newly learned activity.

So if you want to exercise more and your goal is fat loss, muscle building, and a firmer and healthier body, then you must work out consecutively for thirty days. You must eat the right diet and time your meals and your workouts, as well as treat yourself to enough relaxation and regeneration.

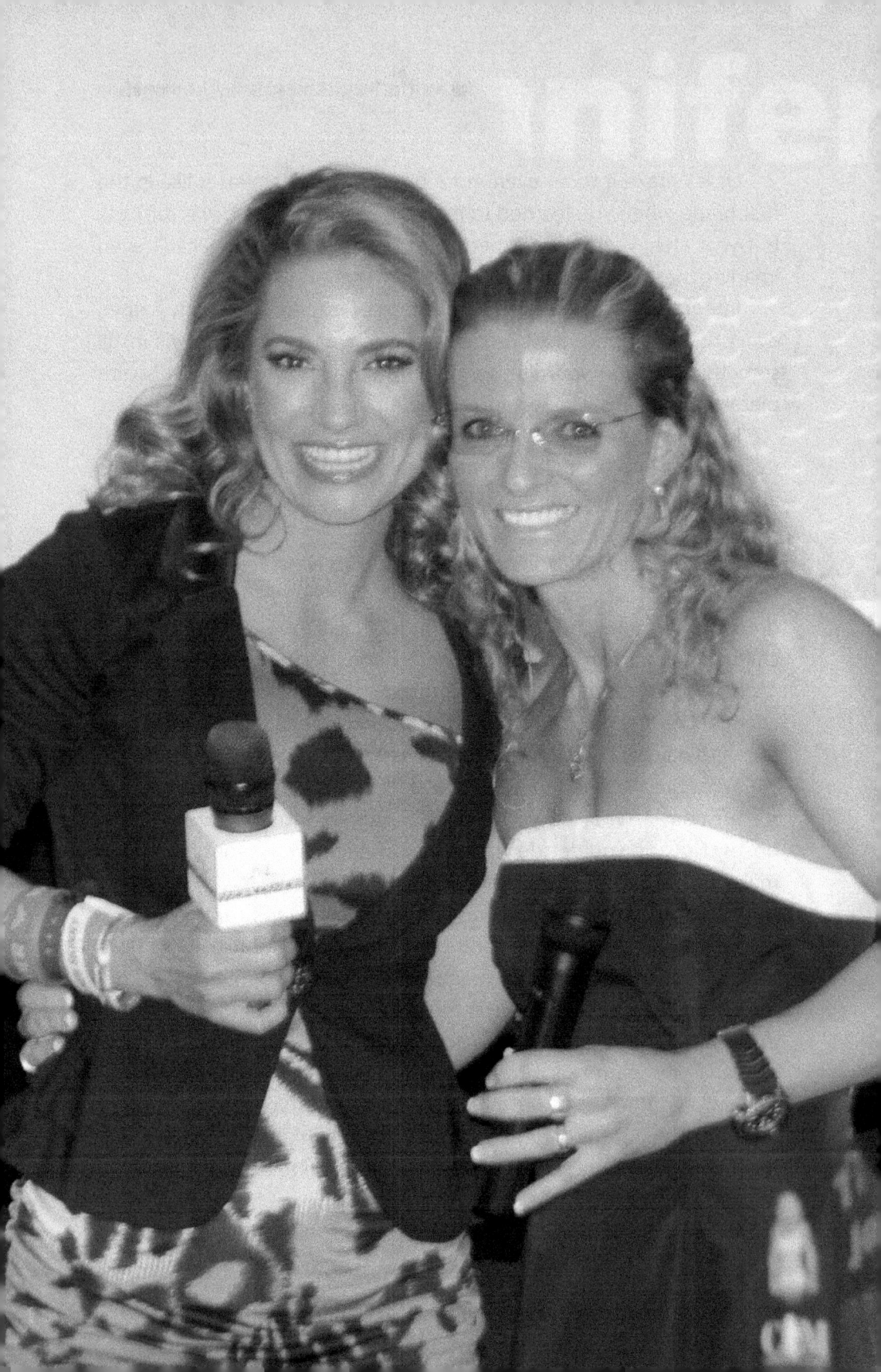

CHAPTER 5

Eat to Blast Fat and Tone Muscle: Your Superstrong and Sexy Body Diet (The Fun, Fit Foodie Plan)

Losing weight is hard enough. Let's make it easy!

In this chapter we will learn how to stop eating accidentally and get off the fad diets. The Fun, Fit Foodie Plan celebrates eating healthy without sacrificing taste. We don't want to diet! If you look at the first three letters of the word "diet," what does it spell? D-I-E! But we don't want to *die*, we want to live, and live optimally. And in order to live a healthy life, we must eat healthy, highly nutritious foods.

Many of us are eating accidentally, eating whatever we stumble upon and finding ourselves getting lunch out of a vending machine. This crazy circus must end by following a food plan. If we plan our food and prepare our meals, we will stick to our plan.

Getting proper nutrition is 70 percent of your success when it comes to getting your ideal body—that's already more than half of your success! How much do fitness models eat, and when? You might be surprised to find they eat plentiful, varied, and anything-but-boring food. This is essential to getting the kinds and amounts of nutrients you need.

- You must eat enough food.
- You must eat a variety of food.
- You must eat exciting food that tastes good!

This is the foundation of the Fun, Fit Foodie Plan. And now we're going to show you how to make it work for you.

Fun, Fit Foodie Sample Meals

First of all, here are some typical sample meals you can eat that are healthy and will help you burn fat. These are a great place to get started and to give you an idea of all the delicious foods you will be eating on this long-term plan.

Breakfast
- Egg-white omelet with veggies and low-fat cheese with a side of whole-wheat toast
- Low-fat milk and fruit smoothie blended with protein powder of your choice (Our favorites are strawberry/blueberry and banana/peanut butter.)
- Smoked salmon with low-fat cream cheese on a small whole-wheat bagel

Midmorning Snack
- Apple with two tablespoons of peanut butter and low-fat, low-sugar yogurt
- Low-fat string cheese with a side of sliced tomatoes drizzled with olive oil and salt-free Italian seasoning
- Nutritional shake

Lunch
- Grilled chicken salad with a small whole-wheat roll or side of whole-wheat crackers
- Blackened salmon with a side of steamed vegetables and brown rice
- Tuna-fish salad made with a touch of low-fat or fat-free mayonnaise on a bed of fresh, crisp greens with a side of whole-wheat crackers or a whole-wheat roll

Afternoon Snack (4:00 or so)
- Handful of almonds (about twelve) and a pear
- Banana sliced lengthwise, smeared with two tablespoons peanut or almond butter, drizzled with honey, and accompanied by a handful of Wheat Thins
- Low-fat cottage cheese with a dollop of sugar-free preserves

Dinner
- Baked tilapia with sweet potato and a side salad
- Seared Asian-seasoned tuna with a side of seaweed salad and miso soup
- Grilled flank steak, sautéed tomatoes, and brown rice with small side salad

Healthy Fast-Food Choices

We all have busy lives with overbooked schedules and demands we can't keep up with. We simply don't have time to julienne red pepper, mince garlic, and defrost chicken! Let's face it: although cooking and preparing meals does have certain bonuses, we can't do it every day. So when we're out in the real world, what do we eat?

With our fail-proof list of dos and don'ts, and what to look for and what to avoid, eating out or eating on the go is a cinch!

What to Avoid
- Fried foods
- Foods loaded with gravies or heavy sauces
- Sugary treats disguised as health foods (granola bars, "snack mix," breakfast bars, etc.)
- Cokes, colas, drinks that pack a whopping two hundred calories per serving
- White bread sandwiches
- Mayonnaise, oil, butter, margarine

What to Look For
- Baked or grilled meats

- Whole-wheat bread or brown rice as a side
- Fresh vegetables and fruits
- Low-fat snack-size servings that are low in sugar (Read the labels! You can't assume it's healthy even if the word "healthy" appears on the label.)
- Low-sodium alternatives
- Olive oil and flaxseed oil

What to Do
- Always ask for no cheese, no sour cream, or no soy sauce on the food you order. (They are loaded with unnecessary fats or sodium.)
- Always ask for sauce on the side.
- Always request whole-wheat or whole-grain bread when given a choice.
- Choose low-fat milk or skim milk instead of half-and-half.
- Ask for grilled instead of fried.
- Ask for water instead of the diet soda or cola that comes with your meal combo.
- Ask for olive oil instead of butter for your whole-wheat bread.

Fun, Fit Foodie Grocery List
Here is a list of superpower foods you should always have in your house. These are the carbohydrates, fats, and proteins that will increase your metabolism and support burning fat and building lean muscle.

Proteins
- Boneless, skinless chicken breast
- Tuna (water packed)
- Fish (salmon, sea bass, halibut)
- Shrimp
- Extra-lean ground beef or ground round (92–96 percent)
- Protein powder
- Egg whites or eggs

- Rib-eye steaks or roast
- Top-round steaks or roast (aka stew meat, london broil, stir-fry)
- Top sirloin (aka sirloin top butt)
- Beef tenderloin (aka filet, filet mignon)
- Top loin (New York strip steak)
- Flank steak (stir-fry, fajita)
- Eye of round (cube meat, stew meat, bottom round, 96 percent lean ground round)
- Chicken, ground turkey, turkey breast slices or cutlets (fresh meat, not deli cuts)

Complex Carbs
- Oatmeal (old-fashioned or quick oats)
- Sweet potatoes (yams)
- Beans (pinto, black, kidney)
- Oat-bran cereal
- Brown rice
- Farina (Cream of Wheat)
- Multigrain hot cereal
- Pasta
- Rice (white, jasmine, basmati, arborio, wild)
- Potatoes (red, baking, new)

Fibrous Carbs
- Green leafy lettuce (green leaf, red leaf, romaine)
- Broccoli
- Asparagus
- String beans
- Spinach
- Bell peppers
- Brussels sprouts
- Cauliflower
- Celery

Other Produce and Fruits
- Cucumber
- Green or red peppers
- Onions
- Garlic
- Tomatoes
- Zucchini
- Fruit: bananas, apples, grapefruit, peaches, strawberries, blueberries, raspberries
- Lemons or limes

Healthy Fats
- Natural-style peanut butter
- Olive oil or safflower oil
- Nuts (peanuts, almonds)
- Flaxseed oil

Dairy and Eggs
- Low-fat cottage cheese
- Eggs
- Low- or nonfat milk

Beverages
- Bottled water
- Crystal Light
- Green tea
- Pomegranate juice

Condiments and Miscellaneous
- Fat-free mayonnaise
- Reduced-sodium soy sauce
- Reduced-sodium teriyaki sauce
- Balsamic vinegar

- Salsa
- Chili powder
- Mrs. Dash
- Steak sauce
- Sugar-free maple syrup
- Chili paste
- Mustard
- Extracts (vanilla, almond, etc.)
- Low-sodium beef or chicken broth
- Plain or reduced-sodium tomatoes (sauce, puree, paste)

Fun, Fit Foodie Recipes

Now it's time to get started with some of our favorite recipes in a convenient meal-plan format.Being a Fun, Fit Foodie, we never have boring, carboard box-tasting meals. We enjoy healthy, balanced meals that make our tastebuds do cartwheels while maintaining our waistline.

Day One Breakfast
Southwest Veggie Omelet
(made with coconut oil)

Ingredients:
- 1 tablespoon virgin coconut oil
- 3/4 cup of your favorite veggies suitable for an omelet (We suggest fresh spinach, mushroom and green pepper.)
- Cherry tomatoes cut in half
- 3 egg whites and one whole egg
- 1 tablespoon skim milk
- Black pepper
- Cayenne pepper

Directions:
1. In a small pan, melt the coconut oil. Add the vegetables and sauté until tender.

2.   Next, add the cherry tomatoes, stir, and sauté for 2 minutes.
3.   While the vegetables are sautéing, beat the eggs with milk in a small bowl. Add black and cayenne pepper to taste.
4.   Pour eggs into the pan and scramble lightly.

Serves 1 to 2. Serve with a slice of low-carb toast, 1/2 cup of prepared old-fashioned oatmeal, or 1/2 cup of high-fiber cereal. You can top your toast with sugar-free preserves and also add some fresh strawberries or blueberries to your cereal.

Midmorning Snack
Vanilla Coconut Protein Shake

Ingredients:
- 1 cup skim milk
- 1 scoop of vanilla protein shake mix
- 1 cup ice (depending on preferred consistency)

Directions:
1.   Blend and serve.

Lunch
Grapefruit Chicken Salad

Ingredients:
- 1 1/2 cups grapefruit segments, cut into bite-size pieces
- 2 cups diced cooked chicken
- 1/4 cup chopped celery
- 1 scallion, minced
- 1/4 cup mayonnaise
- 1/4 cup plain yogurt
- 1/4 cup fresh parsley, minced
- 1 pinch celery seed

Directions:
1. Combine all ingredients and mix thoroughly.
2. Serve on a bed of salad greens and with a side of whole-wheat crackers.
   Serves 3 to 4.

Late-Afternoon Snack
JNL Cayenne Coconut Thai Soup
This delicious soup will hold you over until dinner, and it's been proven that soup fills you up quickly, thus curbing your appetite. Make a whole pot, and freeze individual portions. Bring this soup with you to work and warm it up in the microwave for a hot, delicious snack that will fill you up without filling you with guilt! And it's a great soup to have if you feel a cold coming on. The cayenne helps to fight off fever, and the coconut oil boosts your immune system. This soup is a great addition to the Fun, Fit Foodie Plan.

Ingredients:
- 1 teaspoon coconut oil
- 1 tablespoon unsalted butter
- 1 clove garlic, chopped
- 4 shallots, chopped
- 2 small fresh red chili peppers, chopped
- 1 cup red bell pepper, sliced lengthwise
- 1 cup broccoli
- 1 tablespoon chopped lemongrass
- 2 1/8 cups chicken stock
- 6 ounces lean chicken breast, cut into bite-size chunks
- 1 1/2 cups unsweetened coconut milk
- 1 bunch fresh basil leaves

Directions:
1. In a medium saucepan, heat oil and butter over low heat.

2. Sauté the garlic, shallots, chilies, red bell pepper, broccoli, and lemongrass in oil until fragrant.
3. Stir in chicken stock, coconut milk, and chicken, and bring *almost* to a boil.
4. Simmer on low heat until chicken is cooked.
5. Add some extra cayenne at this point. Make it as hot and spicy as you like!

Dinner
Grilled Grapefruit-Marinated Chicken Breasts with Avocado
Bored with chicken? Not with this recipe!

Ingredients:
- 4 chicken breasts
- 1 pink grapefruit
- 1 navel orange
- 1 lemon
- Lemon-pepper seasoning
- 1 whole avocado, sliced

Directions:
1. Marinate four chicken breasts overnight in a mixture of freshly squeezed grapefruit, lemons, and oranges.
2. Sprinkle lemon pepper on marinated breasts.
3. Heat grill. Grill chicken breasts, being careful not to over- or undercook.
4. For garnish, grill four slices of grapefruit. Top chicken breasts with grilled grapefruit slices.
5. Serve with a side of avocado, a side of brown rice, and a steamed vegetable or salad to make a complete meal.

Dessert
Chocolate Pound Cake with Cappuccino Pudding
The power of cocoa is unquestionable. Cocoa has been shown to:

- Decrease blood pressure
- Improve circulation
- Lower death rate from heart disease
- Improve function of endothelial cells that line blood vessels
- Defend against destructive molecules called free radicals, which trigger cancer, heart disease, and stroke
- Improve digestion and stimulate kidneys
- Treat patients with anemia, kidney stones, and poor appetite

Aim to use the darkest chocolate available, which is 72 percent and can be found at Godiva specialty stores.

Ingredients:
- One large fat-free chocolate pound cake (Entenmann's)
- 1/2 cup extra-dark chocolate (found at Godiva)
- 2 cups light silken tofu
- 1 tablespoon dry instant coffee or espresso
- 1 teaspoon boiling water
- 1/2 cup low-fat sour cream
- 1/4 cup sugar
- 1/4 cup Splenda
- 1 teaspoon vanilla extract
- 1/2 teaspoon cinnamon

Directions:
1. Drain tofu and blend in food processor until smooth.
2. Melt the dark chocolate and add to tofu.
3. Combine coffee with boiling water and add tofu.
4. Add sour cream, vanilla, and cinnamon and blend until creamy.
5. Slice pound cake and place on serving dishes. Add a large dollop of cappuccino pudding.
6. Garnish with large strawberries and slivered almonds if you choose.

Day 2 Breakfast
Fruit Smoothie with Coconut Oil

Start the day off with a breakfast bang! Wash down your vitamins with a rich, delicious protein smoothie thickened with coconut oil. The main differences between virgin coconut oil and refined coconut oil are scent and taste. All virgin coconut oils retain the fresh scent and taste of coconuts, while refined coconut oils have a bland taste due to the refining process.

Ingredients:

- 2–3 tablespoons virgin coconut oil at room temperature (It doesn't matter if is it liquid or solid.)
- 1 scoop vanilla whey protein powder
- 1 cup skim milk
- 3 ice cubes
- Fruit of your choice (whatever you have in the fridge at the time—bananas, blueberries, and strawberries work well.)

Directions:

1. Place all ingredients in a blender or food processor and blend until smooth.

Midmorning Snack
Protein Power Snack

Ingredients:

- 1 snack pack fat-free cottage cheese
- 1 tablespoon sugar-free preserves
- 1 teaspoon coconut oil
- 1 pinch cinnamon

Directions:

1. Swirl sugar-free preserves into cottage cheese (your protein source).
2. Drizzle coconut oil on top and add cinnamon.

Accompany your power protein snack with a side of whole-wheat crackers and a cup of hot green tea, or serve it cold if you wish.

Lunch
Siciliano Protein-Packed Antipasto
This dish makes for an interesting and fun lunch that is just as pleasing to the eye as it is to the tummy!

Ingredients
- Lean cuts of turkey breast
- Black and green olives, rinsed off to rid of excess salt
- Low-fat or fat-free swiss cheese
- Low-fat mozzarella cheese
- Cherry tomatoes cut in half and drizzled with virgin olive oil
- Broccoli florets and carrot sticks
- Pickled banana peppers
- Side of whole-wheat crackers

Directions:
1. On a plate, arrange all ingredients.

Late-Afternoon Snack
Coconut Cookies
They sound sinful—but they're not. They're actually great for you because they are low in sugar and high in fiber from the oats, and the flaxseeds add texture and are a great source of essential fatty acids. What a great guilt-free treat! Add a fat-free, snack-size cottage cheese, and you're set until dinner.

Ingredients:
- 1 cup unsweetened coconut flakes
- 3 tablespoons warm water
- 1 whole egg

- 1 tablespoon honey
- 1 teaspoon coconut oil (for greasing the cookie sheet)
- 1/4 cup flaxseeds
- 1 cup old-fashioned oats

Directions:
1. Mix warm water and honey together.
2. Add the coconut flakes, the flaxseeds, and the oats
3. Beat in the egg. Mix thoroughly.
4. Form into balls and drop by spoonful on well-greased cookie sheet.
5. Bake at 400 degrees Fahrenheit for 12–15 minutes.

Approximate yield: 1 dozen

Dinner
Siciliano (Turkey) Meatballs
One of my favorite memories as a child was sitting around a table enjoying a bowl of spaghetti and meatballs. Now I exchange the high-fat ground beef for low-fat turkey, slashing the calories while keeping the protein high—and they taste delicious! And as for the pasta, use whole-wheat or spinach pasta to up the fiber. Yes, you can have carbs, but the right ones. And watch your portion control. Aim for no more than one cup of pasta and four meatballs.

Ingredients:
- 4 slices of dry whole-wheat bread
- 1/2 cup water
- 2 tablespoons cold-pressed extra-virgin olive oil
- 4 egg whites
- 3/4 cup low-fat parmesan cheese
- 1 pound ground turkey
- 1 tablespoon salt

- 2 teaspoons oregano
- 1 teaspoon parsley flakes

Directions:
1. Leave bread out all day so it is dry.
2. Put bread in bowl and pour water over it. Let the water soak in, then squeeze out excess water and discard.
3. Break up bread with fingers. Add egg whites, parmesan cheese, parsley flakes, meat, salt, and oregano. Mix together with your hands. Taste for salt.
4. Roll into small two-inch balls and put on cookie sheet sprayed with nonstick oil. Bake in a 350-degree oven for 20 to 30 minutes.

Dessert

Grapefruit Tart

Ingredients:
- 2 pink grapefruits
- 1 orange
- 1/2 cup fat-free, sugar-free vanilla pudding
- 8 prebaked sponge-cake shells

Directions:
1. Using a sharp knife, peel rind and pith from grapefruits and orange.
2. Cut into sections and set them aside to drain.
3. Spread vanilla pudding over a sponge cake shell.
4. Arrange drained grapefruit and orange sections over pudding. Serve immediately.

Dessert

Siciliano Tiramisu

This is a super-protein-packed dessert loaded with taste, creaminess, and sweetness—all the things a dessert should have but without the guilt! Extra cocoa powder and delicious, tart strawberries add to the antioxidant punch this dessert packs.

Ingredients:
- 1 large container fat-free ricotta cheese
- 1 tablespoon cocoa powder
- 5 teaspoons instant espresso powder or instant coffee powder
- 1 teaspoon Splenda or Equal
- 1 teaspoon vanilla extract
- 1 teaspoon almond extract
- Sugar-free, fat-free chocolate pudding
- Slivered roasted almonds
- Ladyfingers
- Fresh-cut strawberries
- Fat-free whipped cream

Directions:
1. In a bowl mix the ricotta cheese, cocoa powder, almond and vanilla extracts, and Splenda. Set aside.
2. In a 9-by-9 dessert tray, layer the ingredients as follows: ladyfingers, ricotta mixture, and low-fat, sugar-free chocolate pudding.
3. Top with fat-free whipped cream and garnish with roasted slivered almonds and fresh strawberries.

Special-Occasion Dinner
Appetizer: Roasted Red Peppers in Olive Oil and Garlic with Grilled Shrimp

Peppers are powerhouses packed with an incredible amount of vitamin C, giving you almost 300 percent of your RDA per serving! Shrimp is an excellent source of low-fat, low-calorie protein that is high in selenium, which is needed in small doses for overall health. And everyone knows the wonders of olive oil and garlic! So start your meal off right with this appetizer.

Ingredients:
- 4 large red bell peppers, cut in half
- Olive oil
- 2 tablespoons minced fresh basil
- 2 teaspoons balsamic vinegar
- 1 loaf whole-wheat bread, warmed to a light crisp in toaster oven
- Salt-free Italian seasoning
- 1 clove garlic
- 24 pieces fresh shrimp, peeled and deveined

Directions:
1. Rub the peppers with olive oil and place on a cookie sheet.
2. Broil on high for about 3 to 5 minutes, until you see the skin bubble up brownish black. Take peppers out and place inside a plastic bag (this trick will allow you to take the skin off more easily). When the peppers are cool, rub off skin.
3. Place the peeled pepper in a bowl and add vinegar, Italian seasoning, and basil.
4. Serve on a colorful plate with the side of bread, or place the peppers on top of the bread.
5. In a heated skillet add olive oil and slightly brown garlic. Add the shrimp, cooking 3 to 4 minutes until pink in color.
6. Serve with peppers and bread.

Salad: Barley Vegetable Salad with Feta

Hands down, barley is the best whole grain for you because it carries more fiber than brown rice. One cup of whole-grain barley flour has nearly fifteen grams of dietary fiber and just two grams of fat. Whole-grain wheat has comparable levels of dietary fiber, but the fiber in wheat is almost entirely insoluble. Barley has a very high level of viscous soluble fiber (called beta-glucan)—about 25 percent of the fiber found in whole-grain barley is water-soluble.

Studies have shown that a diet high in viscous fiber such as beta-glucan helps lower blood LDL cholesterol (so-called "bad" cholesterol) levels, a risk factor for heart disease. Such diets may also help stabilize blood-glucose levels, which could benefit people with non-insulin-dependent diabetes.

Whole-grain barley contains high levels of minerals and important vitamins like calcium, magnesium, phosphorus, potassium, vitamin A, vitamin E, niacin, and folate. The vitamin E found in whole-grain barley contains both tocopherols and tocotrienols—powerful antioxidants that research indicates may reduce the risk of certain cancers and help lower blood pressure. Barley is usually used in soups or stews, but I like to use it to "beef" up a delicious vegetable salad sprinkled with feta. Dig in!

Ingredients:
- 1 cup cooked, hulled barley
- 1 cup water
- 1 green bell pepper, seeded and diced
- 1 1/2 cups chopped carrots
- 1 cup red cabbage
- 1/2 cup minced red onion
- 1/4 cup minced sundried tomatoes
- 1 tablespoon red wine vinegar
- 2 teaspoons horseradish mustard
- 1 teaspoon olive oil
- Ground pepper to taste
- 1 pinch cayenne pepper
- 2 tablespoons feta cheese

Directions:
1. Cook hulled barley per directions. Put in a large mixing bowl; add green pepper, carrots, cabbage, tomatoes, and onion.
2. In a small bowl, mix together vinegar, mustard, and oil.
3. Pour over barley mixture and stir to coat.
4. Top with feta cheese. Season with black and cayenne pepper.

Soup: Spicy Winter Squash

Squash is loaded with vitamin C (great for boosting your immune system and fighting off colds) and fiber (to keep your internal functions working regularly). Cayenne is great for circulation, and coconut oil has medicinal properties to fight off infections and thyroid overstimulation. But your family won't even think of how good this soup is for them because of how rich and delicious it is!

Ingredients:
- 3/4 spanish onion, chopped
- 2 teaspoons coconut oil
- 2 1/2 teaspoons curry powder
- 1 pinch cinnamon
- 1/2 teaspoon cayenne pepper
- 4 cups reduced-sodium, nonfat chicken or vegetable broth
- 5 large squash, baked until soft, then pureed
- 1 sweet potato, baked until semisoft and then cubed
- Black pepper
- Topping: fat-free sour cream and whole-wheat croutons

Directions:
1. In a large saucepan, sauté onion in oil for 2 minutes.
2. Add curry powder and peppers, stirring to coat.
3. Add broth and sweet potatoes, and bring to a boil.
4. Reduce heat to medium, partially cover, and cook 7 to 10 minutes.
5. Remove from heat and top with a dollop of sour cream and whole-wheat croutons.

Entrée: Baked Blackened Salmon Steaks with Mango and Black Bean Salsa

Salmon is my favorite fish; it's loaded with omega-3 fat, which is great for our skin and fights off cancer. The only way to get omega-3 fats is to eat them because your body does not make them. The fruit in the salsa adds a kick of sweetness and is loaded with vitamin C. The black beans add fiber and are rich in antioxidants.

Ingredients:
- 1 large mango, pitted and diced into half-inch pieces (1 1/2 cups)
- 1 kiwi, peeled and diced (1/2 cup)
- 15 ounces black beans, rinsed and drained
- 1/3 cup cilantro, chopped
- 2 scallions, sliced
- 2 teaspoons honey
- 1/2 teaspoon salt
- 1/4 teaspoon cayenne pepper
- 2 tablespoons salt-free blackening seasoning
- 1 lime, squeezed with juice set aside
- 4 salmon steaks, 4 ounces each

Directions:
1. Heat oven to 350 degrees.
2. Make the salsa: in a mixing bowl, toss the first nine ingredients with half of the lime juice. Set the salsa aside.
3. Place salmon steaks on a cooking tray and drizzle the remaining juice over the fish.
4. Sprinkle both sides with the blackening seasoning.
5. Bake until cooked through, about 15 to 20 minutes.

Dessert: Grilled Pears and Peaches with Warm Honey Sauce
While pears and peaches are loaded with fiber, walnuts are loaded with omega-3 fat, and blueberries are an antioxidant powerhouse. It would be sinful *not* to eat this dessert because it is just so good for you!

Ingredients:
Honey Dressing
- 1 cup low-fat vanilla yogurt
- 2 tablespoons honey
- 1 tablespoon fresh lemon juice
- 1 tablespoon coconut oil

Topping
- Chopped walnuts
- Unsweetened coconut flakes
- 1 pint of blueberries, washed
- 1/4 cup chopped fresh mint
- 4 ripe pears
- 4 ripe peaches

Directions:
1. Preheat oven to 300 degrees.
2. Whisk the yogurt, honey, coconut oil, and lemon juice in a small bowl.
3. In another bowl, combine the blueberries and mint. Place in fridge until ready to use.
4. Lightly brush pears and peaches with coconut oil and grill.
5. Place grilled fruit in mixing bowl with blueberries and mint. Evenly divide among four plates, drizzle with honey sauce, and top with walnuts.

Fun, Fit Foodie Bonus Recipes
These protein shakes are creative and delicious. Your tastebuds will never get bored! As you know by now, protein shakes are extremely useful in ensuring you get adequate amounts of protein when you are short on time.

Footsteps to Success Iced Chai Protein Shake
Prep Time: 3 minutes

Ingredients:
- 8 ounces water
- 1 scoop vanilla- or chai-tea-flavored whey protein
- 1/2 cup of chai-tea concentrate
- 1 pinch cinnamon
- 1 pinch ground ginger

Directions:
1. Pour water into blender.
2. Add powder, chai-tea concentrate, cinnamon, and ground ginger.
3. Blend on medium speed for 15 seconds.

JNL Fit Tip: If you can't locate chai-flavored protein powder, you can use vanilla flavored. You can usually find chai-tea concentrate in the coffee-and-tea section of your grocery store.

Footsteps to Success Cookies and Cream Protein Shake
Prep Time: 3 minutes

Ingredients:
- 12 ounces cold water
- 1 scoop cookies-and-cream whey protein powder
- 1/4 cup Cool Whip Lite
- 6 ice cubes
- 3 chocolate wafer cookies

Directions:
1. Pour water into the blender. Add protein powder and blend on medium speed for 15 seconds.
2. Add Cool Whip and ice cubes; blend for 30 seconds on high speed. Add cookies and blend on medium speed until mixed.
3. Pour into a tall glass and enjoy.

Footsteps to Success Chocolate Peanut Butter Protein Shake
Prep Time: 3 minutes

Ingredients:
- 12 ounces cold water
- 1 packet chocolate whey protein
- 1 tablespoon natural peanut butter
- 6 ice cubes

Directions:
1. Pour water into blender. Add protein and blend on medium for 15 seconds.
2. Add peanut butter and blend for 30 more seconds. Add ice cubes and blend on high speed until smooth (about 30 more seconds).
3. Pour into a tall glass and enjoy.

CM's Favorite Footsteps to Success Recipes
Here's a collection of my all-time favorite fat-blasting and muscle-fueling recipes.

Breakfast
Blueberry and Vanilla Pancakes

Ingredients:
- 4 large egg whites
- 1 large scoop vanilla whey protein
- 3 tablespoons almond milk
- 4 tablespoons soft oatmeal
- 1 teaspoon wheat bran
- 1/2 teaspoon cinnamon
- 1/2 teaspoon baking powder
- 1/2 cup blueberries
- 1 tablespoon natural Peanut Butter
- 1/2 tablespoon organic honey
- 1/2 teaspoon virgin coconut oil for cooking

Directions:
1. Mix eggs, oatmeal, wheat bran, whey protein, cinnamon, and baking powder in a blender.
2. Pour the mixture into a bowl, cover, and let rest 5 minutes.
3. Heat a nonstick skillet over medium and add coconut oil.
4. Pour the batter into the pan and cook 30 seconds.
5. Sprinkle blueberries over the batter.

6. Turn pancakes after 2 minutes and cook on the other side 2 more minutes until golden brown.
7. Spread peanut butter and honey on the pancakes and serve.

Power Muesli

This is my favorite breakfast when I'm in a hurry but still want to enjoy a powerful and healthy fat burner in the morning.

Ingredients:
- 1/2 cup oatmeal
- 1/2 cup almond milk
- 1 large scoop cookies-and-cream whey protein powder
- 1/2 teaspoon cinnamon
- 1 apple
- 1 tablespoon organic almond butter

Directions:
1. Mix all ingredients; heat briefly in the microwave
2. Top with apple and enjoy

Supereasy Turkey Omelet

Ingredients:
- 3 egg whites
- 1 whole egg
- 3 tablespoons skim milk
- 1/4 pound turkey
- 1 small red onion
- 1 handful fresh baby spinach
- 1 pinch sea salt
- 1 pinch black pepper
- 1 teaspoon extra-virgin olive oil

Directions:
1. Heat the pan on medium heat
2. Pour in olive oil; add diced onions and sauté until translucent.
3. Cut the turkey into strips and cook until a slightly crispy.
4. Whisk eggs and milk together. Pour egg mixture into the pan and sprinkle with baby spinach.
5. Cook on both sides until the light golden brown.
6. Serve on a plate and enjoy.
   Tip: Try with 1 tablespoon low-fat sour cream as a topping.

Easy and Healthy Snacks
These are my favorite snacks, which you can eat with no regrets because you know you're giving your body everything it needs.

You should have two small snacks per day, one between breakfast and lunch and the second in the afternoon.

Green Protein Bomb

Ingredients:
- 2 cups fresh baby spinach
- 1 scoop vanilla whey protein
- 1 tablespoon coconut butter
- 1/2 teaspoon cinnamon
- 1 cup almond milk

Directions:
1. Combine all ingredients in a blender until creamy. Enjoy immediately; if you make it in advance and eat it later, the spinach may get a bitter aftertaste.

Apple with Peanut Butter Rice Cakes and Cottage Cheese
When you need something to grab on the go, this is the perfect snack. It tastes heavenly, and you have filled your body with valuable essential

fatty acids, vitamins, and complex carbohydrates. The cottage cheese gives you protein, and suddenly your energy levels are back up for the day.

Ingredients:
- 1 small apple
- 2–3 rice cakes
- 1 tablespoon peanut butter
- 1 tablespoon organic honey
- 1 pinch cinnamon
- 1/2 cup cottage cheese

Directions
1. Cut apple into slices.
2. Spread peanut butter on the rice cakes. Drizzle honey and cinnamon on top.
3. Serve with apple and cottage cheese.

No-Guilt Midnight Snack
Sometimes there are evenings when I want to cheat so badly! When I have cravings for a full-calorie dessert, this heavenly light cream is worth *more* than its weight in gold.

Ingredients:
- 5 egg whites*
- 1 large scoop whey protein (any flavor)
- Cinnamon (to taste)
- 1 teaspoon almond butter

Directions:
1. Put egg whites, whey powder, and cinnamon in a blender and mix on high about 5 minutes, until fluffy and creamy.
2. Immediately pour into a bowl. Drizzle more cinnamon and almond butter over it and enjoy immediately.

*Please pay attention to the quality of eggs you buy, and always store them in a cool place so that you need have no fear of salmonella. Use only eggs from free-range hens that are not corn fed; you can eat these eggs raw without worry.

Turkey Red Pepper Boats

This recipe is so easy to make, and a delicious source of high-quality lean protein.

Ingredients:
- 1 red bell pepper
- 1/4 pound turkey
- 1 cup cottage cheese
- 1 pinch of pepper
- Salt-free seasoning

Directions:
1. Cut the pepper in half and scoop out the seeds, making two "boats."
2. Dice turkey and mix with cottage cheese.
3. Fill the pepper boats turkey/cottage cheese mixture and season with pepper and seasoning.

Whole-Wheat Toast with Cocoa, Honey, and Almond Butter

Ingredients:
- 1 slice whole-wheat bread
- 1 tablespoon almond butter
- 1/2 tablespoon organic cocoa powder
- 1 tablespoon of organic honey
- Cinnamon to taste

Directions:
1. Toast bread.

2. Mix almond butter and cocoa and spread on the toast.
3. Top with honey and cinnamon for a superpower snack!

Lunch
Turkey Muffins

This is a perfect to-go lunch for taking to the office or on a trip. It is absolutely delicious, kids love it, and there's no mess involved.

Ingredients
- 1 pound turkey breast, cut into cubes
- 3 tablespoons Parmesan cheese
- 3 stems rosemary
- 3 cloves of garlic, cut or crushed
- 1 cooked and quartered sweet potato
- 1 egg
- 1 teaspoon or less sea salt
- muffin tray, preferably silicone

Directions:
1. Preheat oven to 350 degrees. Blend all ingredients in a food processor.
2. Brush muffin tray with olive oil and remove extra oil with a paper towel. Fill each muffin cup with dough.
3. Bake in the oven 30 minutes. Allow to cool a few minutes before taking the muffins out of the mold.

Serve with 1 percent yogurt, low-fat sour cream, or organic no-sugar-added ketchup as a dip.

Turkey Bowl with Fresh Veggies

Ingredients:
- 1 pound turkey breast, cut into cubes
- 4 large tomatoes
- 1 medium onion, chopped

- 1 zucchini, cut into half moons
- 1 eggplant, cut into cubes
- 9 mushrooms, sliced
- 1 red bell pepper
- 3 cloves garlic, sliced or crushed
- 10 basil leaves, chopped
- 2 tablespoons fresh parsley, chopped
- 1/2 teaspoon sea salt
- 1 tablespoon cold-pressed olive oil

Directions:
1. Heat oil in a large frying pan or wok and sauté the turkey cubes until lightly brown.
2. Add onions and cook until translucent; set turkey and onions aside in a separate bowl.
3. Add remaining ingredients and cook 15 minutes over medium heat until the vegetables are al dente.
4. Return the meat to the pan and simmer briefly before serving. Serve with a small bowl of brown rice or whole-wheat pasta.

Here are some more options I love for quick, fit, and healthy lunches.
1. Make up a big salad bowl of fresh veggies such as baby spinach, broccoli, kale, zucchini, and cucumber, dressed with balsamic vinegar, extra-virgin olive oil, and lemon juice vinaigrette and topped with some lean protein like fish, beef (organic and grass-fed), turkey, or chicken. On the side, have some whole-grain bread, couscous, or brown rice.
2. Fill whole-grain wraps with scrambled egg whites and veggies.
3. A clever option for a low-carb version of spaghetti noodles is shirataki or konjac noodles—they have no carbs and no calories! Yes! Really! Shirataki noodles are made largely of water and high-fiber konjac flour; they have hardly any flavor, and therefore can absorb other flavors, such as tomato sauce. Top with a sauce made of ground beef,

tomatoes, some more veggies, olive oil, and some salt-free season-ing. You really can eat as much as you like, and there are no carbs!

Dinner
Kale Rolls with Tomato Zucchini Sauce

Ingredients:
- 1 1/4 cup ground beef
- 1 egg
- 4 large kale leaves (about 1/2 cup)
- 1/4 cup low-fat mozzarella
- 1/2 bunch parsley
- 1/2 cup tomatoes
- 1/2 cup zucchini
- 1 cup of water
- 1 pinch black pepper
- 1 pinch salt

Directions:
1. Briefly cook the kale leaves in hot water and remove the coarse stems.
2. Chop parsley and grate mozzarella.
3. Mix meat, mozzarella cheese, parsley, and pepper together in a bowl.
4. Spread kale leaves with the meat mixture and roll up.
5. Place the rolls in a baking dish and pour in 1 cup water. Bake for 15 minutes at 350 degrees.
6. Cut zucchini into thin strips and mix with the tomatoes, basil, sea salt, and pepper to make sauce.
7. Take the rolls from the oven. Pour the sauce over them and bake for an additional 15 minutes.

Grilled Squid with Garlic Sauce and Feta-Stuffed Pepper

Ingredients:
- 1 1/2 cup squid

- 1 lemon
- 2 cloves of garlic
- 1/2 cup low-fat yogurt
- 1 tablespoon olive oil
- 1 red bell pepper
- 1/3 cup feta cheese
- 1 egg
- 1/4 cup sour cream
- 1 pinch black pepper

Directions:
1. Cut off the top off the pepper and carefully scoop out the seeds with a knife.
2. Cut the feta cheese into small cubes; place in a bowl and mash with a fork.
3. Mix sour cream, egg, and black pepper. Scoop the mixture into the pepper.
4. Place the stuffed pepper in an ovenproof dish and bake at 350 degrees for about 30 minutes.
5. In the meantime, sprinkle the squid with lemon juice and olive oil, and grill until thoroughly cooked.
6. Mince the garlic and mix well with the yogurt in a bowl.
7. Serve the grilled squid with the pepper and drizzle with garlic sauce.

Dessert

These great little dishes are all very healthy and can be eaten without guilt. They are so delicious and are great for your soul and body.

Mini-Carrot Cupcakes with Frosting
Makes 12 minicupcakes.

Ingredients:
Cupcakes
- 1/2 cup carrots, peeled and cut into chunks + 3 tablespoons water

- 1/2 cup flaxseeds
- 1 cup almond flour
- 1/2 teaspoon baking soda
- 1/3 teaspoon sea salt
- 1 teaspoon cinnamon
- 1/4 teaspoon nutmeg
- 1/4 teaspoon ground ginger
- 3 tablespoons maple syrup (more if you like)
- 2 tablespoons coconut oil, melted
- 1 egg
- 1 teaspoon pure vanilla extract
- 1/4 cup golden raisins
- 1/4 cup chopped walnut or pecans
- 1/4 cup unsweetened, shredded coconut

Frosting
- 1/3 cup low-fat cream cheese
- 2 tablespoons coconut butter
- 3 tablespoons organic honey
- 1/4 teaspoon pure vanilla extract

Directions:
Cupcakes
1. Preheat oven to 350 degrees and line a minicupcake pan with twelve liners.
2. Steam carrots in a pan with some water until soft, checking every few minutes to see if they are ready.
3. Place carrots and cooking water in a food processor and puree.
4. Combine almond flour, flaxseeds, baking soda, salt, cinnamon, nutmeg, and ginger in a bowl.
5. Stir together maple syrup, coconut oil, egg, and vanilla in another bowl.
6. Mix wet ingredients into the dry, and then fold in carrots, raisins, nuts, and shredded coconut.

7. Divide batter among muffin tins and bake 16 to 20 minutes or until set in center.
8. Remove to wire rack to cool.

Frosting

1. In the bowl of a stand mixer or with a handheld electric mixer, beat together cream cheese, coconut butter, honey, and vanilla until incorporated and fluffy.
2. Frost cupcakes when they have cooled.
3. Store in fridge.

Chocolate Walnut Brownies

These are not just for adults—they're also big hit at kids' parties!

Ingredients
*   1/2 cup unsweetened baking chocolate
*   1/2 cup organic whole grain sugar
*   3 egg whites
*   2 eggs
*   2 tablespoons coconut butter
*   1/3 cup applesauce without added sugar
*   1 teaspoon real vanilla extract
*   1 teaspoon cinnamon
*   3 teaspoons cocoa powder
*   1/2 cup whole-grain spelt flour
*   1/2 cup walnuts
*   1/2 teaspoon baking powder

Directions
1. Preheat oven to 350 degrees.
2. Melt baking chocolate in double boiler or pot on low heat, then set aside.
3. Mix eggs, sweetener, applesauce, coconut butter, and cinnamon in a bowl.

4. Whisk together flour and baking powder. Stir into egg mixture, then add melted chocolate and nuts.
5. Pour batter into a parchment-lined flat cake pan.
6. Bake in the oven for 30 to 35 minutes.
7. Allow to cool before cutting into squares and serving.
   Makes 9 brownies.

Superdelicious Zucchini Cake

Ingredients:
- 1/2 cup organic whole grain sugar
- 4 egg whites
- 1 egg
- 1/2 cup applesauce without added sugar
- 1 teaspoon cardamom
- 1 teaspoon cinnamon
- 2 tablespoon coconut oil
- 1 cup grated zucchini
- 2 cups whole grain spelled flour
- 1/2 teaspoon sea salt

Directions:
1. Preheat oven to 350 degrees.
2. Mix eggs, sweetener, applesauce, and spices in a bowl.
3. Whisk together flour and baking powder, and add to wet ingredients, mixing thoroughly.
4. Pour batter into a loaf pan and bake in the oven about 50 minutes.
5. Allow to cool and remove from the pan.

Date Almond Energy Bars

Ingredients:
- 1 1/4 cups quick oats

- 3 tablespoons whole-wheat flour
- 1/3 cup wheat germ
- 1/2 cup slivered almonds
- 1/2 teaspoon cinnamon
- 1/2 teaspoon sea salt
- 3/4 cup whole pitted dates, chopped
- 1/4 cup honey
- 1/4 cup olive oil
- 1/4 cup almond butter

Directions:
1. Preheat oven to 350.
2. Line an 8-by-8 pan with parchment paper so that it folds up and comes out two sides of the pan.
3. In a large bowl, mix together oats, flour, wheat germ, almonds, cinnamon, and salt. Mix in the dates.
4. In another bowl, thoroughly whisk the honey, olive oil, and almond butter.
5. Pour the wet ingredients into the dry and mix well.
6. Spread the batter into the prepared pan and pack firmly.
7. Bake for 20 to 25 minutes or until brown at the edges.
8. Remove from oven and let cool for 15 minutes. Using the overlap of parchment, lift bars out of pan.
9. Place on a rack and cool completely. Cut into 12 squares.

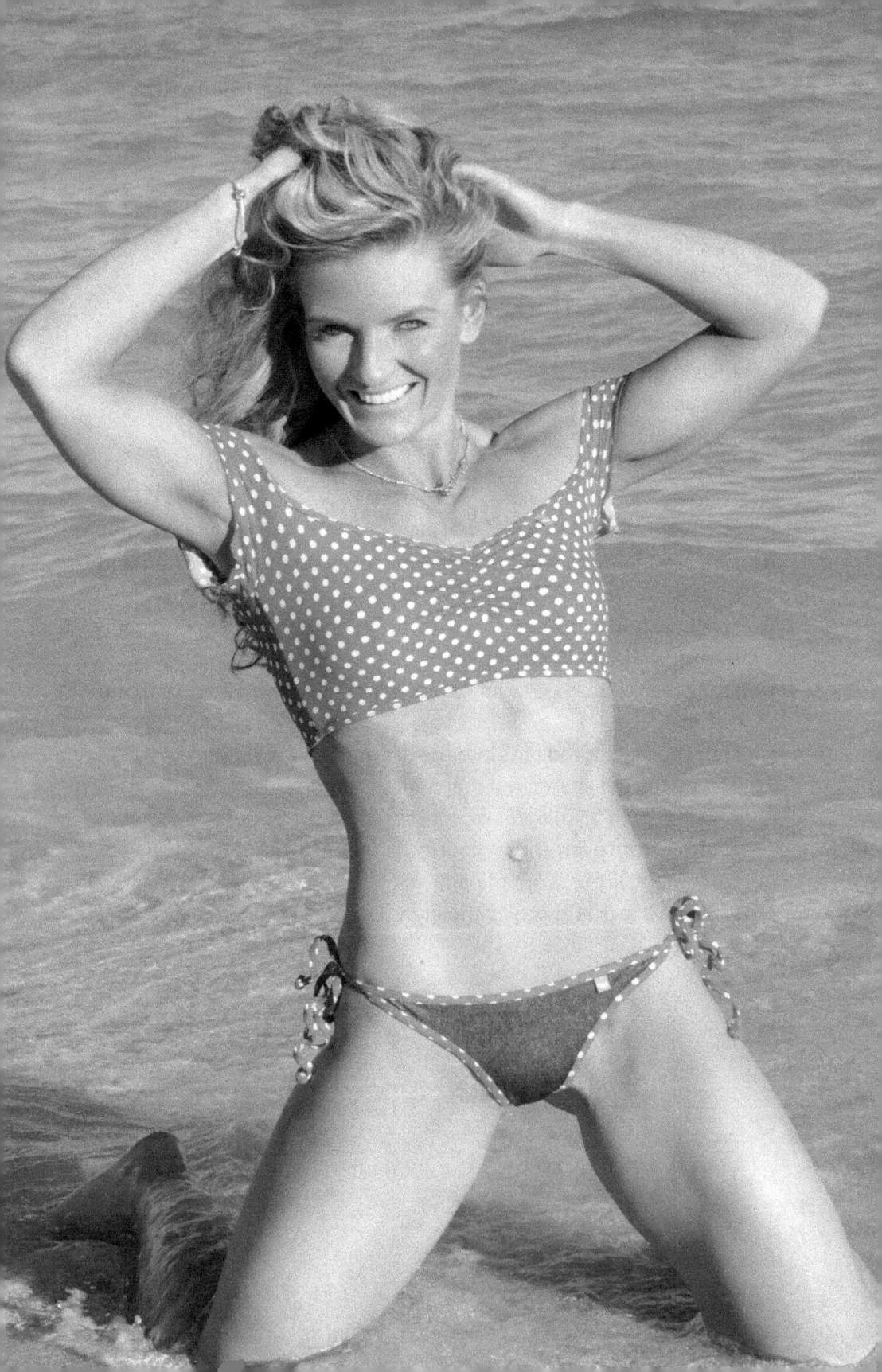

CHAPTER 6

Burn, Baby, Burn! Best JNL Fusion
Workouts to Blast Fat and Tone Muscle

The Footsteps to Success lifestyle program is based on the principle that muscle tissue burns more calories than fat tissue, therefore increasing metabolism. When a person's metabolism is increased, it makes it easier to burn fat and keep it off forever. To gain muscle, you must strength train, provide the growing muscle with sufficient protein, and rest.

Ask any doctor, cardiologist, personal trainer, or licensed nutritionist why some people burn off fat more quickly than others. The unanimous answer is their metabolism! Metabolism can be defined as the rate at which we burn off calories. Our metabolism rate is, unfortunately, inherited. However, fortunately enough, this is where our fat-blasting principles will help you to increase your metabolism and lose weight. We will give you the necessary tools and steps to actually stoke your metabolism, turning your body into a roaring furnace that burns off the fat even when it's at rest. These steps in combination with healthy habits in general will allow you to finally "crack your weight-loss code" and unlock your weight-loss and fat-burning potential.

Once you begin the Footsteps to Success lifestyle program, you will experience an "aha!" moment. You will realize what it takes for your body to release the fat you've been storing for years.

Cracking the Code to Your Metabolism

Losing weight only to gain it back and constantly seeing the number yo-yoing up and down on the scale made me (Jennifer) feel just like a hacker who sits at a computer for hours, days, or maybe even weeks, attempting to crack into a protected site. How frustrated I got! I had the motivation and the drive to lose weight, but I was like a gerbil on a wheel going nowhere fast. I tried all the fad diets and exercise gadgets. I looked in my closet and found clothes ranging from size 0 to size 16. I said to myself, "This can't be right!" I looked in my bathroom: three scales, a fat measurer, a tape measure, and a mirror where I would daily judge my appearance.

Then, I looked into my bedroom. I found the same scenario. I found weights, an elliptical machine, a jump rope, and the latest, hottest weight-loss gadgets—you name it, I had it. Did all these gizmos work? No! My weight still went up and down!

But remember, from chaotic events in our life come great things. I kept on "hacking" my body, trying to find the right method to do three simple things: lose fat, gain muscle, and increase my energy level!

I am proud to say that I did it, and now it's my turn to give you the same tools to help you achieve these same weight-loss results, too!

In this simple plan there are no Band-Aid approaches. We will take you straight to the root cause of why some people store fat and some people burn it off by just sitting at their desks. We've said it before and we'll say it again: the key is their *metabolism*.

We're not going to waste your time. We would like to introduce you to a proven way to increase your metabolism right off the bat: you must increase your lean muscle mass. It's simple math. To add muscle, you must follow this tried-and-true weight-loss-success formula: weight train and then fuel the growing muscle with a proper nutritious food plan that is based on moderate-to-high levels of protein, fiber-rich carbs, and good-for-you fats.

It may seem as if we're stepping out on a limb here and doing something crazy, but *exercise is mandatory* to take true Footsteps to Success. Some of the top-selling diet books state that exercise is nonessential to losing weight. What a lie! I (Jennifer) have even read a top-selling book authored by a cardiologist who stated that exercise is a choice, not a solid part of cardiovascular wellness and physical fitness. Where did he get his degree?

Medical research will show you that all forms of exercise, whether it be a brisk walk or a superduper power-pump session in the gym, are beneficial to the cardiovascular system and for the entire body. You *must* treat exercise in this program like an important business meeting with your body that you cannot miss or be late to.

Exercise is just one of the sequence of numbers that will help you crack the code to your metabolism. There will be no codependency on group meetings or weekly gatherings, and you won't have to buy premade and preprocessed food. Furthermore, you will not have to slave away in your kitchen finely shredding orange peel and peeling/deseeding/slicing papaya for your next "Chicken Raspberry Spinach Salad." This is definitely not the case with our Footsteps to Success lifestyle program. This book is for the everyday busy person who multitasks, and now with these codes to fitness success, you will able to get maximum results with small but smart amounts of effort! You will see maximum results in minimum time.

First of All, What Is JNL Fusion?

I (Jennifer) am honored to say that I have created one of the world's most popular and powerful workout methods to date. JNL Fusion has been called the "workout of the millennium" due to it "fusing" both cardio and strength exercises together in one efficient and effective thirty-minute workout. JNL Fusion is a mix of the most efficient exercise genres including kickboxing, karate, plyometrics, and body sculpting to provide you with a sizzling hot body and results that are noticeable immediately.

I have worked for over a decade in order to create the best, most effective, and fastest way to get you in shape. This program revolves around thirty-second bursts of exercise, called "superspiking," which is all about strength and cardio training infused together. This will take your muscle to the max.

Superspiking works because you are building ripped, lean muscle that your body needs to burn fat all day long, which takes "afterburn" to a whole new level. With this unique superspiking method, you won't get big and bulky; you will get toned and tight!

The basic characteristics, benefits and features of the JNL Fusion workout are listed below:

1. Workouts are time efficient, typically consisting of thirty to forty-five minutes in length.
2. Workouts always follow the pattern of six circuits consisting of three sets of thirty-second strength movements, followed immediately by one of JNL Fusion's signature trademark cardio bursts.
3. Workouts can be adapted for all fitness levels: beginner, intermediate, and advanced.
4. Workouts are designed for both men and women, young and old.
5. You get the best of both worlds with this workout, blasting off ugly fat while revealing sleek, sexy, athletic muscle tone.
6. You don't have to be an athlete to train like one with the JNL Fusion workout.
7. You never overtrain since JNL Fusion systematically trains the right muscle groups at the right time.
8. JNL Fusion has the "yin and yang" of cardio and strength in one complete, time-efficient workout.
9. Workouts can be enjoyed in a limited amount of space.

10. You can get the body of a super fitness model with sexy muscle tone, low body fat, sexy "kiss-me abs," and "glutes that salute"—a body that looks like it jumped off a fitness magazine cover!

What Makes JNL Fusion Different?

JNL Fusion is different from many other workout methods because of many reasons. Instead of doing weight training followed by cardio, the cardio bursts of thirty seconds are woven right into the strength-training workout. I took my experience from my personal weight-loss success story and from years of being in the bikini and fitness competition circuit to create a succinct, dialed-in, and efficient workout method that can be done anywhere—from the gym to your home, backyard, or any outdoor area.

The main characteristics of the JNL Fusion workout method are what make it so simple for anyone—from a beginner to a personal trainer or fitness enthusiast—to choreograph their own JNL Fusion workouts. Also the creative cardio-burst exercises that include inversions are a key characteristic of what makes JNL Fusion different.

Why JNL Fusion Surpasses Other Methods

JNL Fusion has not only been recognized internationally as a superior workout method: it's a workout method that benefits *you* individually for a number of reasons, whether you've been working out with other methods or have just started to exercise.

First, the exercises can be performed in a small space with very little equipment, only a jump rope, a timer, and set of dumbbells. There's little to no learning curve, and the superspiking allows you to get the maximum benefits in the minimum amount of time.

Athletically, JNL Fusion pushes you by training your body's full spectrum, not just in a linear way such as on a treadmill. This helps you embrace your true athletic potential and systematically create the super-fitness-model-body physique. Because of this 360-degree approach, JNL Fusion is designed to produce symmetry in the body, not a boxy silhouette with no waistline. Instead it focuses on pulling in the waistline while adding roundness to the glutes, strength to the legs, and the coveted "fitness model body." "Tight and tiny" athletic and lean muscles are created due to the low-weight and high-rep and bodyweight exercises combined with the superspiking cardio bursts.

This method also increases your endurance, stamina, and athletic capability with plyos, drills, and superspiking cardio bursts. But don't worry—safety is always first, and JNL Fusion is safe for all age levels. With the JNL Fusion philosophy, you're never subjected to unwanted peer pressure to overtrain, outperform, overpush, injure, or exhaust yourself with an unhealthy state of exercising. There are no illogical, random exercise sequences that may lead to overtraining, overdeveloping, or injury.

Instead the JNL Fusion workout method and culture is one of embracing *you* at your current fitness level and helping you safely gain more endurance, stamina, and athletic capability in a fun, nonjudgmental way.

Those who have embraced and used this method have enjoyed gaining lean and athletic muscle tone while blasting off ugly fat. Many "skinny-fat" people have enjoyed gaining sleek, sexy muscle tone, endurance, more energy, and stamina. Remember, it's not the number on the scale that determines if you are fit or not. It's how strong and fit you feel. And strong is the new skinny!

JNL Fusion Workout Accessories
You may want to make a small investment in the workout accessories listed below:

- Gymboss timer—available at www.JNLGymboss.com
- Speed rope
- Cordless jump rope
- Hand weights
- Dumbbells

- Floor mat
- Stability ball
- Long bar
- Ankle weights (optional)
- High tops (optional)—to prevent injury and provide superior support of feet, ankles, and joints when doing plyometrics, jumping rope, etc.

Are you ready for your first JNL Fusion workout?

JNL Fusion Workouts to Blast Fat and Tone Muscle

Get "glutes that salute" and "kiss me abs," and represent that strong is the new skinny! Here are some of the best JNL Fusion workouts for you to enjoy. All you need is a small space, a pair of dumbbells, a jump rope (or cordless jump rope), a thirty-second timer, and a matt for floor work.

Follow the simple formula of six circuits that blend strength with cardio.

JNL Fusion Ab-Ripper Session
WARM UP
Speed Rope (5 minutes)
CIRCUIT ONE
Crunches
Beginner Crisscross Squat (hands on hips)
CIRCUIT TWO
Twist Crunches
Beginner Crisscross Squat (fingers touch the floor)
CIRCUIT THREE
Bent-Knee Leg Raises
Speed-Bag Shuffle
CIRCUIT FOUR
Firecracker Abs
Side Kicks

CIRCIUT FIVE
Standing Twists
Horse-Stance Karate Punches
CIRCUIT 6
Ab-Circle Pro or Ab Roll-Up with Twists
Horse Stance with Torso Twists
COOL DOWN

JNL Fusion Sexy and Sweaty Shoulder Shredder and Triple Tricep Threat
WARM UP
Speed Rope (5 minutes)
CIRCUIT ONE
Shoulder Press
JNL Fusion Burpee
(burpee with a plyo jump to the opposite direction)
CIRCUIT 2
Side Raises
Fusion Jumping Jacks
CIRCUIT 3
Upright Row
Basketball "Shoot for the Hoops"
CIRCUIT 4
Tricep Extension
X Push-Up with a Twist
CIRCUIT 5
Tricep Kickbacks
Tricep Wood-Chop Squat
CIRCUIT 6
Tricep Dips
Fusion Soccer Kicks (go for the goal!)
COOL DOWN

Quick Fitness Tips for Your Everyday Lifestyle

As we are all very busy, especially us moms, here are some simple tricks to help you enjoy a more fun, fit day.

- Speed-bag shuffle first thing after getting out of bed.
- Take the stairs, not the elevator.
- When brushing your teeth, perform alternating knee raises.
- Burn off calories when playing with your kids. When they are little, play Hide and Seek, Catch Me If You Can, and Duck, Duck, Goose.
- When cooking, perform squats.

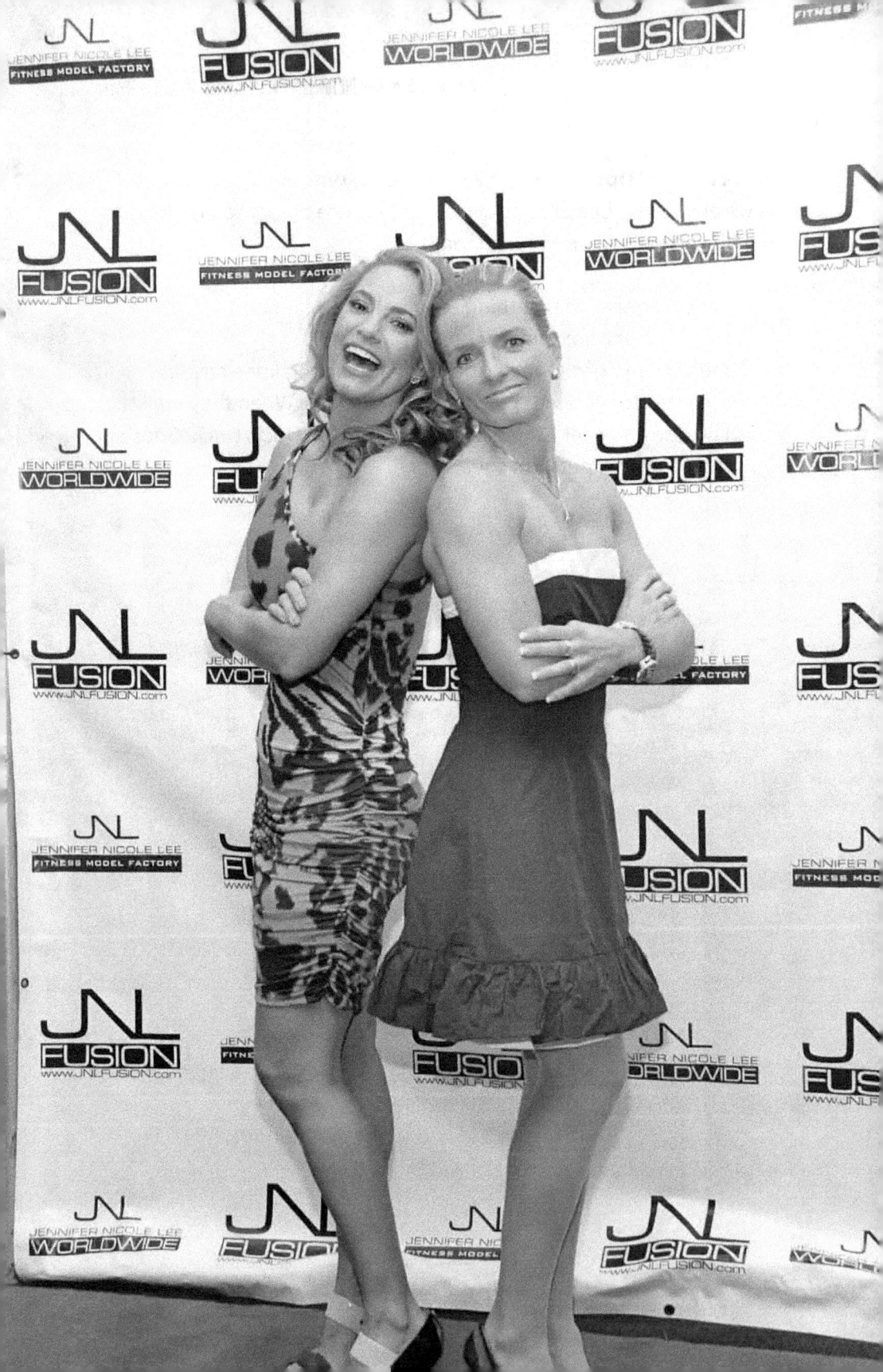

CHAPTER 7

How to End the Self-Sabotaging Behavior of Yo-Yoing and Control Your Appetite

You've already learned so much in this book. You're now ready to say good-bye to those fad diets in favor of your new, fit lifestyle. Soon, you'll be loving your newfound dream body. There's no reason to be afraid of the yo-yo effect anymore!

Let's go over it one more time: out of frustration and ignorance, you probably started one (or more than one) of the "superdiets," which you can find in every women's magazine. For weeks you endured the deprivation; you kept to the diet plan and might have even made it through ambition and discipline to your destination weight. However, you could never keep to that goal; after a few weeks or months, the pounds were back, often more than before. And you became afraid of this yo-yo effect before starting any new diet.

But now things are different. You've learned a lot about the right attitude, the focused mind, a new way of eating, and how to exercise. There is no failure anymore because you have the knowledge that makes you sure of your path and equips you for coping with setbacks. Remember, setbacks *belong* on your path and are quite human and natural.

We all have not only highs in our lives but also lows. It's good to know they are coming and be prepared for them so that you come back up faster than you thought you would.

You should know what type you are:

- Are you a "frustration eater" during emotional lows, or do you almost forget to eat when you are experiencing anger and frustration?
- Are you an extremist, thinking "more is better" and exerting yourself until you're completely exhausted?

If you know how you react during these emotional lows, it's much easier to deal with them, and you can beat the yo-yo effect. If you are a frustration eater, it's particularly important to pay attention in difficult times to staying on your diet and eating according to plan. Prepare food in advance, before you have to choose what you'll be eating, and store it in the refrigerator. Try to make these meals so delicious that you won't be tempted to eat anything else. One of my favorite tricks is to already have healthy foods prepared in the refrigerator that I can eat without feeling guilty. This is a fantastic way to trick your inner demons.

If you forget to eat during emotional difficulties, it is particularly important that you prepare your meals in advance and then remind yourself to eat at regular mealtimes by setting an alarm. This will help you avoid slowing your metabolism down so that it burns too little. You will have no more cravings and will find your way back up faster than before.

"More is better"—this is something we have heard all too often! It's anything but effective and can make all your efforts for nothing. Exercise and the right diet should be balanced and take place in the right amounts; otherwise, you're working against your own body. You need regeneration times to replenish your body. If your body is in balance and gets everything it needs, it is working optimally and also burning more than if you were exerting it until it was on its last legs.

It's not about being perfect, it's about being persistent. Aim to work out four to five days a week. On days that you know will be very busy, make this your off day from working out. Make sure you schedule your down time as well. Enjoy a nice bath or a relaxing walk. You will be more prepared for the next day and have more energy for your next workout.

In short, preparation is the best medicine!

We know this from our own experience that it can sometimes be difficult, but when you're prepared, a few mistakes are no big deal. Plan your work, then work your plan. If you know what to do in advance, you will be setting yourself up for success.

And the nice thing is that every day you can jump on the fit and healthy train again. Each new day is ready for a new decision, so use this opportunity!

Here are our top tips for good preparation against setbacks:

1. Always have healthy snacks prepared so that when you have a ravenous hunger attack you'll have something to reach for other than chocolate or potato chips.
2. Cut up bite-sized fruits and vegetables, and prepare a delicious sweet dip of low-fat cottage cheese, vanilla, and organic peanut butter or a savory dip of low-fat cottage cheese, chili powder, sea salt, and herbs.
3. Try something new! Choose foods from our list in chapter 6, and make your favorite meals and snacks. Don't be shy about having fun with the recipes, especially to create something new. You'll see that it will be worth it.
4. Begin to know your body and find out when and what situations cause an unwanted craving attack. Is it due to an annoying emotional situation? Or are you rewarding yourself with a certain food? Remember, we are all products of our past and are preprogrammed by previous thought patterns and situations.

One great way to reward yourself instead is with a fantastic workout. This does your mind and body more good than eating something unhealthy, and you'll feel even better afterward. You won't feel guilty—you'll feel proud that you reached your goal.

So if you're eating out of frustration, put on your workout clothes and train instead. A forty-five-minute JNL Fusion workout, and your anger will be forgotten! You'll look and feel like new, for you have transformed your anger and frustration into pure power and energy.

No matter how much preparing you do, you may have short periods of time when things are not going so well and you put on a few pounds—but that's not bad! Because you know now how weight loss actually works, you can repeat your exercise habits and improve your consistency at any time.

So don't be afraid to make mistakes—they are part of the game! Don't condemn yourself for unintentional slip-ups—you're human and it happens. Ultimately you won't even notice these occasional mistakes if your basic diet is based on healthy, fresh, and unprocessed foods.

Starting today, you can banish the yo-yo effect from your life! You have more than enough strategies in your toolbox to fight it if it briefly appears. Enjoy your new life and your new dream body without fear.

Outsmart the Cravings Monster: How to Control Your Appetite
Another way to end the vicious cycle of yo-yoing is to control your appetite. But we must learn how to control our appetites by controlling our emotions. When we get emotional, this triggers eating for comfort, not for nutrition.

Do you feel that sometimes you are ruled by inner demons urging you into the kitchen to gorge upon endless amounts of packaged cupcakes? Do you sometimes feel that your body is being possessed and controlled by something forcing you to eat food that you shouldn't be touching? Do you sometimes find yourself in your pantry eating sugary sweets, high-calorie treats, and high-carb snacks?

We all experience the strong desire for food, the urge to eat, and the unquenchable appetite that can be boiled down to one word: *craving*! It's human nature, and we all have dealt with the forceful passion to eat foods that are on our "do not touch" list. So how do we get a firm hold on our cravings? Can we think differently, behave differently, even exercise and eat differently to place a harness on our sometimes-out-of-control appetites? How can we hold off this human urge to eat things we should not really even be thinking of? What triggers cravings, and how can we fight them and win?

Your cravings and appetite are out of control because you are most likely not on a fitness program. In our Footprints to Success program, you learn how to eat, train, supplement, and beautify like a true athlete. This program teaches you to outsmart the cravings monster!

The great news is that there are indeed things you can do to manage cravings, even if you can't stop yourself from thinking about the foods you love.

Unlike the everyday normal hunger that we all feel, cravings are the strong yearnings for certain foods that seem to be linked to our mind's reward system. Emotions, uncomfortable situations, or pleasant associations (for example, your mom rewarded you with vanilla ice cream and a handful of animal crackers if you did all of your chores when you were little) can trigger a craving.

It's true that when you eat a food you long for, your brain releases dopamine, a natural chemical related to pleasure. Even the powerful senses such as our senses of smell and sight can trigger a full-on craving episode.

So what do you do the next time you start longing for an entire meat-lover's pizza or a banana split when you're already stuffed from lunch? The following stay-sleek strategies will boost your ability to just say no and keep your sense of peace about food. These tips are also important for those who are preparing for a photo shoot, a competition, or a special event.

JNL's Natural Appetite Suppressant #1: Your "Before" Photo
This is your personal rewind button, and you don't want to push this button at all! In order to know where you're going, you must know where you are currently. And no matter what your fitness level and weight you are now, we urge you to take a "before" photo if you haven't already.

This photo is a powerful visual that will remind you of your weakness and what you need to address and work on. Place it somewhere you will see it every day, reminding you of your soon-to-be past.

This Was Me Then; This Is Me Now!
Some months after I (Jennifer) gave birth to my second son, I took my famous "before" photo and went on a mission to become my healthiest. But I started my own weight-loss journey, and I did not see any results. I was two and a half months into it, and still no real results! I almost gave up and threw in the towel. But a little positive, self-loving voice inside my head told me not to quit and to carry on. Even if I didn't see the results I wanted, I would still benefiting from a superhealthy lifestyle.

Then *it* happened!

A week later, it was as if my body started responding drastically to my new, healthy lifestyle! The fat floodgates finally opened, allowing my body to release the fat it had stored for years, and my muscle mass started to show!

To hear my personal story in depth with all the details, and to really get to know me, please click below. This story will inspire you to never give up and to keep your momentum in life.

https://www.jennifernicolelee.com/JNLSHOP/10Expand.asp?ProductCode=54

So just as I kept at it, I urge you also to never give up when you feel at times like you want to! Use your "before" photo to remind you of what you are working to leave behind.

JNL's Natural Appetite Suppressant #2: A Little Goes a Long Way

Now this is our kind of news: recent research from a major university revealed that surrendering to a craving is sometimes the best course of action—as long as you can practice PC, short for "portion control." In a study of thirty-two overweight women, all averaged an 8 percent weight loss after twelve months, but those who were most successful gave in to their cravings occasionally. When they did indulge, they ate small amounts—just enough to be satisfied.

The main point here is practicing restraint and moderation, not deprivation. When you forbid a food, it only becomes that much more attractive and appealing, and you become likely to overeat.

So when you need to feed the chocolate monster, reach for a pre-packaged snack, such as those cool "100 Calorie Packs" of Doritos, and call it a day. You'll be much less likely to break down and attack an entire plate of nachos with the works.

JNL's Natural Appetite Suppressant #3: Daydream!

Being told to think of something else when you're in the grip of a powerful craving is about as helpful as being told to stay alert when you're fainting. But there is one way that this information can actually help: researchers at a major university in Australia found that occupying your senses with a vivid nonfood daydream just might suppress your urge. Your short-term memory has limited storage.

To conjure any image—nachos or that spring break in Cancun—you need to pull them out of your long-term memory, the way an iPod cues up one song at a time from the gazillion it has in storage. But short-term memory has only so much room; it can't play "Cheeseburger in Paradise" and "Holiday" at the same time. The idea is to keep your short-term memory busy by fantasizing about something else.

This technique has worked for my www.clubjnl.com weight-loss clients. When they were asked to drum up remembered smells and sights—the scent of freshly cut grass or a log fire, and images such as the Goodyear Blimp or the Eiffel Tower—their cravings for cookies (which were right in front of them) were reduced by about 30 percent. Their minds couldn't handle the craving and the new sensory imagery at the same time, so the craving got discarded.

How about this one: try thinking about what your guy or girl looks like in nothing but a towel—you might forget all about that cookie.

JNL's Natural Appetite Suppressant #4: Become a Concoction Queen

No one has ever made a longing for a slice of double-cheese-and-pepperoni pizza disappear by gnawing on carrot sticks. But that doesn't mean healthy substitutions never work. It's all about satisfying your appetite and pleasing the palate. The secret is to get the flavor and texture that you want with the least caloric damage.

If you can't stop thinking about that slice of pecan pie, try baking a sweet potato and blending in some dry oatmeal, pecans, a touch of cinnamon, and brown sugar. Viola! A healthy version of a piece of "pecan pie" with all the nutrient benefits and none of the sugar! Another tip is to try frozen bananas dipped in chopped walnuts instead of a Popsicle, or frozen grapes instead of sorbet. Just be creative.

My weak spot is for nachos, so instead of going to town, I use baked chips with low-fat cheese and reduced-fat sour cream. I also use fat-free refried beans. It's just as good as the real thing, and maybe even better because you are saving so many calories when you get creative. Sometimes you have to reinvent your favorite dish to save your diet.

JNL's Natural Appetite Suppressant #5: Accept That You Are Human and Cravings Happen

Playing mind games isn't the only way to fight the war on cravings and win. If you simply acknowledge your craving, accept it, and choose not to act on it, you have weakened its power over you.

When you're struck by the hunger for that huge plate of fettuccini alfredo, practice cognitive dissemination. Instead of trying to ignore the craving, admit to yourself that you want that big plate of cheesy pasta. It works on the same principle as getting the hots for a coworker when you're in a great relationship: recognizing that you'll always be attracted to cute guys or girls (or yummy food) prevents you from acting on the feeling every time it comes up.

JNL's Natural Appetite Suppressant #6: Use a Visual Cue

Set yourself up for success by always keeping positive visual cues around you. I urge all of my weight-loss clients to keep their momentum, even on their bad days, by having their skinny jeans hanging up in their closet in plain sight. You can also use a bikini you want to wear, a midriff top, or any other visual cue.

I use this story often to illustrate the point that even the masters need to be visually stimulated to take action. Arnold Schwarzenegger would often walk around with a short cut-off shirt on to allow him to always see his stomach and abs area. He knew what he was doing, as it served as a constant reminder to always be on his A-game and to work out and eat right. Use this same technique that works for you to keep your eye on your prize.

JNL's Natural Appetite Suppressant #7: Create a Support Team

Create an inner circle of your closest friends, your personal coach, or a family member you can turn to. Tell them of your weight-loss goal and how you will look to them to help you fight your cravings. One tool I coach my clients on is to have a "Craving Jar." Every time you let a craving get the best of you, you will be held accountable by putting something in the jar. You can set the dollar amount, but make it high enough that it's painful to break.

When I started on my weight-loss program, I made my husband make me pay ten dollars into a jar every time I went over my "cheat-treat" quotient. This technique made me open my eyes to my eating habits and was also extremely helpful in retraining my pregnant eating habits after I had my sons. I needed to make drastic changes, and this really helped! I was forced to give my craving money away, and this taught my taste buds fast.

JNL's Natural Appetite Suppressant #8: Work It Out
Yes! I said a workout. Try this: the next time a huge craving sets in, go for a walk. Get your blood going and your mind off this treat that is haunting you. Get up and get moving! Pretty soon momentum will set in and your craving will be a thought of the past.

Try my JNL Fusion workout method. You will love the strength training and cardio combination in these effective and time-efficient workouts. I offer live interactive workouts online at_www.JNLFitnessStudioOnline.com.

All you need is a webcam and Wi-Fi. Also, there are new, fresh, never-seen-before workout videos you can instantly download and enjoy anywhere and anytime right at www.JNLFitnessStudioOnline.com.

So you see, there are no excuses! Just log on and we will train together.

JNL's Natural Appetite Suppressant #9: Physically Remove Yourself from the Temptation
Not to get "biblical" here, but even the Good Book states that sometimes temptation is so bad and so strong that the only choice we have is to physically remove ourselves from the temptation. I use this technique when I'm at my son's friend's birthday parties. I love cake, so I make it a point to be on the other side of the room engaged in a friendly conversation, especially if I'm dieting down for a competition.

JNL's Natural Appetite Suppressant #10: The Power of Visualization
See yourself in your dream body, in your dream outfit, saying "no thank you" to the food you're craving. Imagine that a server brings it to you

on a plate, and confidently, without a flinch, you turn this meal down. The more you visualize saying no and winning in this scenario, the stronger your willpower and determination to stick to your weight-loss goals will become!

We sure hope that these craving killers will help you achieve your fitness goals, help you to retrain your behavior, and also recondition the way you look at food! Achieving your weight-loss accomplishments is not about perfectionism but persistence. Please also remember that as the saying goes, "Rome wasn't built in a day." So go slowly, and enjoy the process and journey of living a superfit and -fun lifestyle.

For more great resources, please visit:

- www.jnlbooks.com
- www.getfitwithjnl.com
- www.fitnessmodelprogram.com
- www.bikinimodelprogram.com
- www.101thingsnottodo.com
- www.shopjnl.com
- www.jennifernicolelee.com

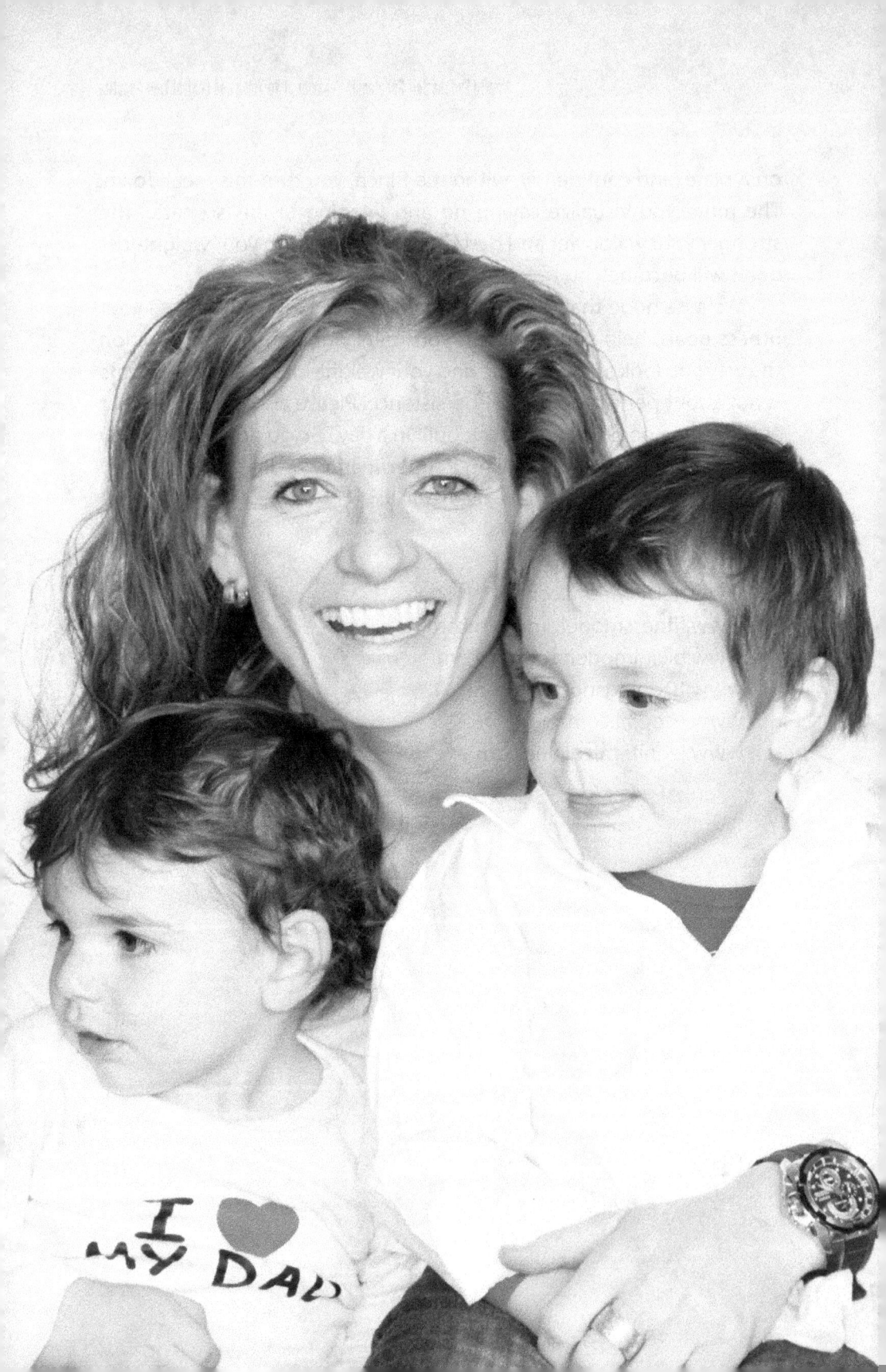

CHAPTER 8

Family-Centered Fitness! JNL Fusion for the Entire Family

You might have been thinking up until now that it's going to be difficult to integrate your new healthy lifestyle and fitness program into your family life. However, it's actually very simple, and that's what we want to show you in this chapter.

Your family is not an obstacle to fitness—in fact, just the opposite, because as a mother you are probably already running around all day, always on the move. Children keep us in motion and give us so much joy in life, and they want to move and be active all day!

Show them how they can help you:

- Train with your children together in the living room. JNL Fusion is 100 percent suited to you *and* your children, and your husband will love it because it is not only very effective but it also makes you feel good!
- Make working out a game by coaching your own boot camp. Teach your kids the individual exercises, and explain to them what to do for each muscle group. This is such fantastic training

for them, and your children will be educated, athletic, and fit from the beginning. It is so much easier to grow up with a good habit than to learn it in later years.

- Spend lots and lots of time in the great outdoors with your family, hiking, riding bikes, and taking trips to forests and lakes to show them how beautiful life can be when we enjoy nature. Being able to spend this time with our children and teach them the important things in life is a gift from God. Have fun with your family and get moving!
- Play a question-answer game about healthy foods that make us strong and fit.
- Cook along with your family. Look at healthy cookbooks and select a meal to prepare together. It's wonderful for children to learn how to prepare unprocessed foods. Let them try anything, for example, cutting some raw vegetables into small slices and others into strips and then tasting them both to see if the flavor changes with the form.

It's so wonderful when children are already growing up with healthy habits. It is our responsibility to our children to share this knowledge, because then we give them one of the greatest gifts: the opportunity to realize their infinite potential, because in a healthy body lies a healthy and clever mind, and the other way around as well.

Let's work together to make the world a little bit better by starting with our families. Each family is a part of our society, and when more and more families are healthy and strong, then those around us can also become stronger, healthier, and happier.

We have a responsibility to make our community stronger, and thus our world, by shaping our children into a new, strong, healthy, and mentally stable generation. Our children are the future of our world, and we must give them the best start possible, as this is the only world we have.

We look forward to making the world a little better with you as our children grow up to be strong and healthy together!

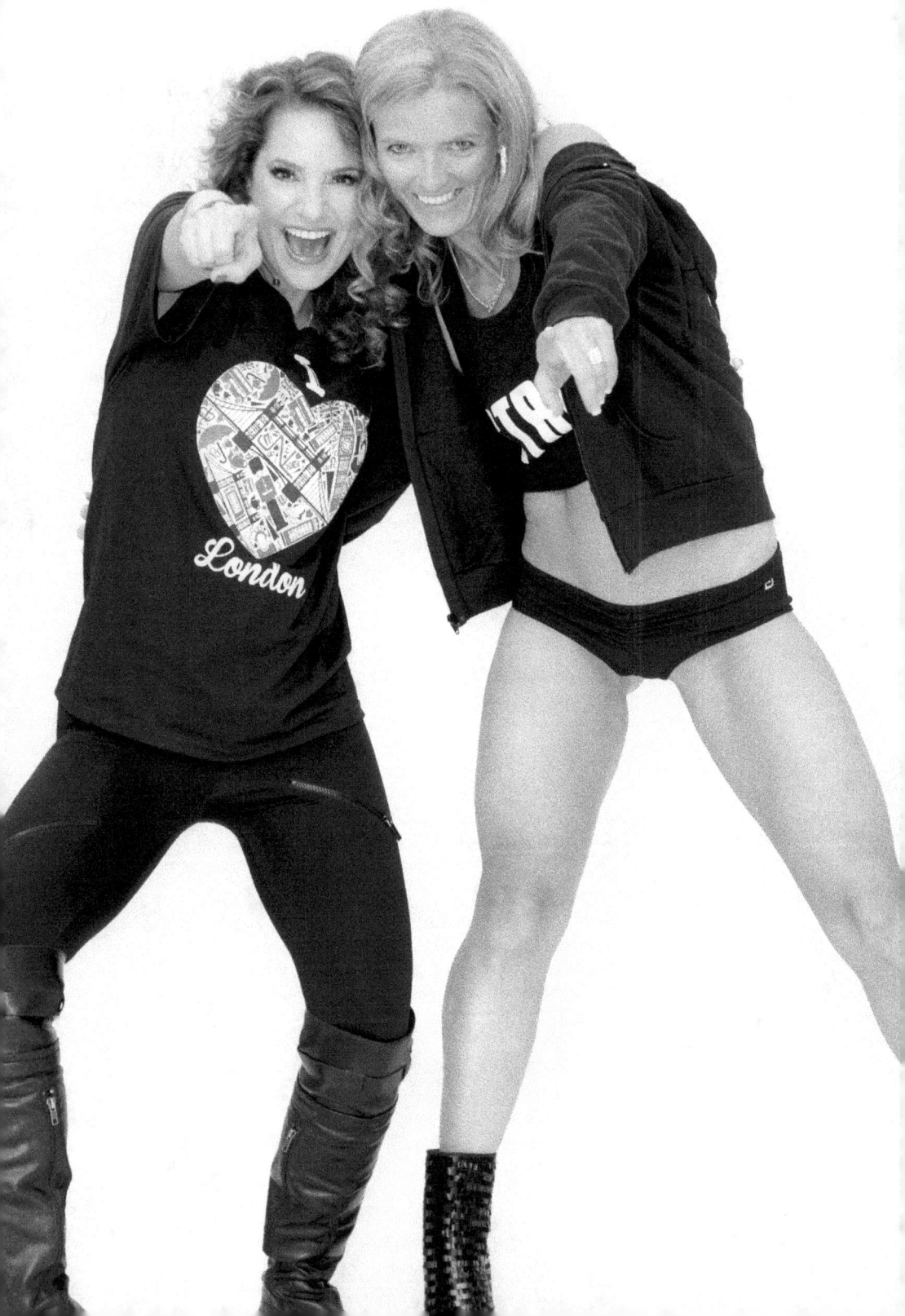

CHAPTER 9

Top Tips and Secrets from JNL and CM

Finally, we would love to provide some final very important tips that should accompany you on your entire journey—not only to achieving and maintaining your dream body but also in all other levels of your life and success.

1. The best strategy is to prepare daily.
If you prepare yourself well in advance, then you have less errors to fix and improve.

To achieve your goal, it's important to first have a plan and then to prepare. Your plan for your dream body should include meal planning and preparation, workout plans, relaxation, and what to do when unexpected things happen—at least until you've internalized your new routine.

Take one or two days per week to cook your meals for the rest of the week. Prepare as much as possible beforehand, and restructure your refrigerator and kitchen so that it's as easy as possible for you to access the food you'll be eating. This will cost you a bit of time, but then everything will be done in just a few hours a week instead of having to do it every day. Then you can begin to better plan and prepare for other important everyday activities.

This approach will simplify your life and your diet so much. Try it and be amazed! With good preparation you will win you a lot of free time, which you can invest in yourself and your family.

2. Put yourself at the top of your to-do list.
You're the most important person in your life! So you should also treat yourself. Your daily to-do list should contain you at the top: your diet, your workout, time for you and your priorities each day—and at least one hour for unforeseen things that might come up.

Plan exercise into your daily schedule as an important business appointment so that it is very hard to cancel. If this should ever be the case, then you can push your exercise time into that extra hour.

Do this so you'll continue to pursue your goal and stay focused. Without a planned and fixed schedule, it is virtually impossible allow for new things every day. Review chapter 4 to help you work out a suitable plan.

3. Give your best every day.
If you get up in the morning with the intention that you will do your best today and it is a great day, then you have created the best conditions for a good day of your own making.

Sometimes we take on too much at once. We want to finish a project, but by the end of the day we might not have succeeded. However, if we give our best every day, this isn't a bad thing.

Often too many unforeseen things come up that interfere with our daily schedule, no matter how much we have planned ahead. This is normal and human. If it happens, don't get annoyed or discouraged but be sure to acknowledge what you *have* accomplished, and be proud of what you've done.

Every night write out a list of things that you have to do the next day on a notepad or, even better, in a note-taking program on your smartphone. This will remind you every day of your goals.

With time, you will be able to optimize your day more and more—despite the fact that you have taken on new activities such as exercise and meal planning.

Be proud of yourself every night that you've gotten one day closer to your goals!

4. Think big and take small steps.

Thinking big is an ability all highly successful people share. Sometimes they think so big that it may seem completely implausible—but they always prove the opposite!

You need a grand vision of you and your life that you're striving for every day and can give your best effort to.

In order to achieve this great vision, you have to first of all believe in yourself.

Believe in You and You Will

If you have found your life vision, break it down to an annual plan, a monthly plan, and finally a weekly schedule. From this you can make the best of every single day, day after day.

This may sound exhausting, but it is anything but! It is incredibly thrilling, exciting, and motivating at the same time, and you always have your vision within you. You have a commitment to yourself to implement your vision so that it becomes reality, which will give you unimaginable strength and energy.

When I (Carolin) discovered Jennifer's weight loss success story on the Internet, suddenly I had found my vision!

I wanted to be like her; I wanted to live life like she did and for my children have a role model like that in me. Since then, I've carried this great vision with me, and it motivates me every day. Throughout my weight loss journey, I used her success story and pictures to motivate me in my day-to-day life. This vision has changed my life completely, and I'm now living my personal dream.

What I can do, you can do, too! Dare to think big and build your very own huge vision. Your life will change completely, and you will turn your vision into reality.

In Closing

We thank you for reading this book! May it help you achieve your fitness and weight-loss goals. Always know we are here for you and you can always reach out to us.

Make sure you also join the number-one online fitness community at www.JNLMethod.com.

We are a strong, happy, healthy, and fun fitness family, and we invite you to share all that you have learned in this book.

We believe in you!

Jennifer Nicole Lee and Carolin Mildner

www.jnlmethod.com
www.jennifernicolelee.com
www.carolinmildner.com

www.ingramcontent.com/pod-product-compliance
Lightning Source LLC
Chambersburg PA
CBHW070926270326
41927CB00011B/2744